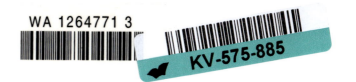

Arterial Stiffness
and Pulse Wave Velocity
Clinical Applications

Roland ASMAR

Review Committee:

Michael O'ROURKE

Michel SAFAR

Foreword by:

Michael O'ROURKE

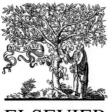

ELSEVIER

Amsterdam, Lausanne, New York, Oxford, Paris, Shannon, Tokyo

A member of Elsevier Science

Roland Asmar, M.D.
L'Institut CardioVasculaire
21, boulevard Delessert
75016 Paris, France

Michael F. O'Rourke, M.D.
The University of New South Wales
St Vincent's Hospital
Darlinghurst NSW 2010, Australia

Michel Safar, M.D.
Service de Médecine Interne 1
Hôpital Broussais
96, rue Didot
75674 Paris cedex 14, France

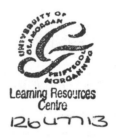

Imprimé en France par STEDI, 75018 Paris
Dépôt légal : 6307-Novembre 1999 ISBN 2-84299-148-6

Printed in France

CONTENTS

Acknowledgements

This book is the author's expression of great acknowledgment for the contribution of our predecessors who, despite limited technical possibilities, have during the nineteenth century developed the recording of the pressure wave and the concept of the pulse wave velocity.

The author acknowledges for his/her appreciable collaboration each of the persons who has introduced him to arterial hemodynamics, supported him in his scientific approach and collaborated in the realisation of his principal studies:
G. Amah, A. Benetos, J. Blacher, P. Boutouyrie, A.M. Brisac, O. Crisan, J. Duchier, X. Girerd, S. Haddad, C. Hugue, P. Lacolley, N. Lahlou, B. Laloux, P. Laurent, S. Laurent, B. Levy, G. London, J.J. Mourad, B. Pannier, M. Safar, F. Sayegh, J. Topouchian, J. Toto-Moukouo, S. Voscorian.

This publication has been made possible through an educational grant of the SERVIER RESEARCH GROUP.

Foreword

With heightened interest in isolated systolic hypertension as the major antecedent factor in cardiac failure, and with the present focus on pulse pressure rather than mean pressure, clinical attention is swinging from peripheral resistance to large artery stiffness, from the smallest arterioles to the largest arteries.

Arterial stiffness is a new concept to many clinicians, even though clinicians and clinical physiologists at the turn of this century established its importance, and developed methods for its measurement.

In this book, the first to specifically focus on arterial stiffness in clinical practice, Prof. Roland Asmar has done a splendid job in reviewing older concepts and blending these with the new work that he and his colleagues have been conducting over the past two decades, and contributions from around the globe.

The focus of the book is on pulse wave velocity, the first and still the best method for measuring arterial stiffness. In major epidemiological studies, pulse pressure is emerging as more important than systolic or diastolic pressure in predicting cardiovascular events. Pulse wave velocity is likely to be found an even better marker of arterial disease and of prognosis.

Prof. Asmar's book is a superb synopsis of the present state of the art.

Michael O'Rourke

Indices of Arterial Stiffness Terminology

■ **'Distensibility'** refers to the capacity and ease of distension.

■ **'Stiffness'** and **'Rigidity'** mean the opposite of distensibility.

■ **'Elasticity'** is used to quantify 'distensibility'.

■ **Capacitive compliance** = relationship between pressure fall and volume fall in the arterial tree during the exponential component of diastolic pressure decay.

$$\Delta V / \Delta P \ (cm^3 \cdot mmHg^{-1})$$

■ **Compliance** = absolute changes in volume following changes in pressure. Compliance represents the slope of the pressure/volume relationship.

$$C = \Delta V / \Delta P \ (cm^3 \cdot mmHg^{-1})$$
where ΔV = change in volume and ΔP = change in pressure

for one unit of length, volume = cross-sectional area depending on diameter, thus:

$$C = \Delta D / \Delta P \ (cm^3 \cdot mmHg^{-1})$$
where ΔD = change in diameter and ΔP = change in pressure

■ **Distensibility** = relative volume or diameter changes for a given pressure change

$$\Delta V / \Delta P \cdot V \ (mmHg^{-1})$$
where ΔV = change in volume, ΔP = change in pressure, V = baseline volume

for one unit of length, volume = cross-sectional area, depending on diameter, thus:

$$Distensibility = \Delta D / \Delta P \cdot D \ (mmHg^{-1})$$

■ **Elastic Modulus (Peterson)** = the inverse of distensibility; ie, the pressure changes required for a (theoretical) 100% stretch (wall pressure for 100% diameter increase)

$$EP = \Delta P \cdot D / \Delta D \ (mmHg)$$

■ **Oscillatory compliance** = relationship between the oscillating pressure change and oscillating volume change around the exponential pressure decay during diastole.

$$\Delta V / \Delta P \ (cm^3 \cdot mmHg^{-1})$$

■ **Pulse wave velocity** = speed of travel of the pulse along an arterial segment distance

$$PWV = Distance / Time \ delay \ (m \cdot s^{-1})$$

■ **Stiffness index (β)** = ratio of log (systolic/diastolic pressures) / (relative change in diameter)

$$\beta = \ln(P_s/P_d) / [(D_s\_D_d)/D_d]$$

■ **Strain** = Δl / l

   where l = *length at baseline,* Δl = *change in length for a given stress*

■ **Stress** = P × R / h (mmHg)

   where P = *transmural pressure,* R = *radius and* h = *wall thickness*

■ **Young's elastic modulus** = wall tension per centimeter wall thickness for 100% diameter increase

$$E = \Delta P{\cdot}D \ / \ h{\cdot}\Delta D \ (cm^3{\cdot}mmHg^{-1})$$
where h = *wall thickness*

Young's modulus represents the slope of the stress–strain relationship.

CHAPTER

Introduction and historical overview

INTRODUCTION

Cardiovascular disease is the leading cause of mortality in most industrialised populations. Large-artery pathology is the major contributor to cardiovascular disease morbidity and mortality. The initiation and progression of the pathological functional and structural alterations in large arteries such as arteriosclerosis are only partially understood. In addition, given the insidious nature of most of the cardiovascular risk factors and the arterio-atherosclerotic processes, early recognition of arterial changes and lesions (functional and/or structural) may help us to identify individuals with a high risk of clinical complications. Thus, the potential public health benefit derived from a more complete understanding of the etiological role of arterial lesions in cardiovascular disease or its utility as a risk marker for preclinical arterio-atherosclerosis is considerable [1-3].

Historically, large arteries were considered to be passive conduits of blood, involved only in blood transport and distribution. More recently, several studies have shown that large arteries constitute a complex and fully functional organ with conduit and distribution functions (and also endocrine and paracrine functions) as well as a blood pulsatility buffering capacity. The latter mechanical properties of the large arteries are important determinants of circulatory physiology in health and disease; elastic large arteries absorb energy during the systolic component of pulsatile flow and thereby reduce the cardiac work for a given cardiac output. The study of large-artery dynamics is inherently difficult, due to the pulsatile nature of blood flow, the complex structure of the vessel wall and the continually changing tone of the smooth muscle component. Several methods are now employed to evaluate the structure and function of the large arteries [4-7].

Invasive methods

Such methods as angiography or other imaging techniques allow a precise evaluation of the arterial lumen or an analysis of the arterial wall structure. Their use is complex, expensive, and requires very sophisticated technical equipment, which restricts their application in large clinical trials.

Noninvasive methods

These are based mainly on ultrasound techniques (high-definition ultrasonography, duplex echo-Doppler, 'Echo-Tracking') and computer analysis of the video signal and/ or ultrasound signal to study the function and/or structure of some arterial axes and sites accessible through these methods. These relatively sophisticated techniques remain reserved to some clinical research laboratories [7-10].

Of these noninvasive methods, the measurement of pulse wave velocity (PWV) is one that has been widely employed for a long time to evaluate arterial wall distensibility and stiffness. This method is noninvasive, simple, accurate, and reproducible, thus it can be easily applied in large therapeutic and epidemiological studies [11-14]. The general purpose of this book is:

    – to explain arterial stiffness, pulse wave velocity (PWV) and its principles;

    – to describe the methods of its measurement;

    – to analyse its determinants;

    – to investigate its clinical implications in terms of pathophysiology, diagnosis, prognosis and therapy.

HISTORICAL OVERVIEW

Before the examination of the arterial pulse as a hemodynamic parameter of blood circulation, philosophers, physicians, anatomists, and embalmers strove towards an explanation of pulse wave physiology. Many centuries before Christ, the Egyptians described the pulse wave as the 'word' of the heart to the vessels; later on, the Chinese analysed the quality of the pulse, and its examination took on the form of a mystic rite. For them, an ample and prominent pulse was considered as a positive and healthy sign, while a hypokinetic or weak pulse described weakness. Thus the pulse amplitude was used as an index of vivacity, vigour and health. According to legend, Chinese sphygmology was founded by the Emperor Hoamti, who is said to have been the author of several books on the pulse about 2500 BC, and to have been very skilled in the art. After the patient's arm had been placed on a cushion, the pulse was palpated in three separate places by the physician's index, ring and middle fingers, respectively. At each site, light, moderate and firm pressure was applied in turn so as to elicit the superficial and deep pulses. The various pulses were represented by symbols like the jump of a frog, the tail of a fish, drops falling on a roof, and so on. The use of pulse diagnostics is today still a part of traditional Chinese medicine. At the time of Hippocrates (460–377 BC) and Aristotle (384–322 BC), the relation between the pulse and the heartbeat was not recognized, and the arteries were considered to contain air and to communicate with the trachea. Later on, Galen (131–200 AD) was the first to note a relationship between the heart and the arteries and pointed out that the arteries contain blood and not air. He ranks as the foremost sphygmologist of antiquity, not merely because he wrote a number of books on the subject, but because his teaching on the pulse dominated clinical practice for about 16 centuries. He recognized that the arterial pulse was dependent on and synchronous with the heart, but he believed that the artery possessed its own pulsatile or sphygmic faculty. The variations of the pulse due to age, sex, season, country, sleep, pregnancy, exercise, etc., were described at length.

The first attempt to represent the pulse graphically, in a form comparable with a sphygmographic tracing, was made by Struthius in 1540, who studied the pulse wave by placing a leaf on the artery and watching its vibrations.

It was only in 1553 that Miguel Serveto (1511–1553) described the pulmonary circulation and in 1628 that William Harvey (1578–1657) described the circulation of the blood. Harvey's work established the pulse wave as a manifestation of cardiac ejection, stressed that cardiac systole corresponds to the arterial diastole, and considerably improved comprehension of the arterial pulse and its clinical applications. More than 100 years later, in 1731, the Reverend Stephen Hales (1677–1761) recorded the first invasive arterial pressure measurement. During the 18th and 19th centuries, the theories of fluid and wave transmission were established and Etienne Marey (1830–1904) was the first to accurately record the arterial pulse in man using a sphygmograph *(figure 1)*. The introduction of the sphygmograph and later of arterial pulse and blood pressure

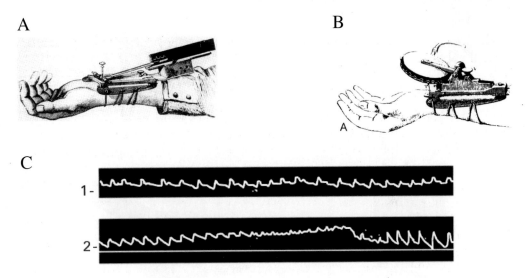

FIGURE 1. Sphygmographs of E.J. Marey (1830–1904).
A. Mechanical sphygmograph. B. Air-filled transmission sphygmograph. C. 1 - Respiratory variability of the pulse. 2 - Variability of the pulse characteristics during and after an exercise test.

recording into clinical medicine marked the beginning of the arterial hemodynamic approach *(figures 2–6)*. The introduction of the Riva Rocci brachial cuff and sphygmomanometer in 1896 and the description of the Korotkoff sounds in 1905 allowed the measurement of the maximal (systolic) and minimal (diastolic) values of the pressure pulse and thus led to the disappearance of the sphygmographs and of pulse wave analysis from clinical practice *(figures 7, 8)*. Despite this simplistic and incomplete approach to the pressure wave, physicians began to record the systolic and diastolic blood pressure because they were simple to determine, and left pressure wave analysis to experts in cardiology and vascular conditions [15, 16].

The pulse wave, as a diagnostic tool, has attracted people for several thousand years. It is generally agreed that a high percentage of all cardiovascular disorders is associated

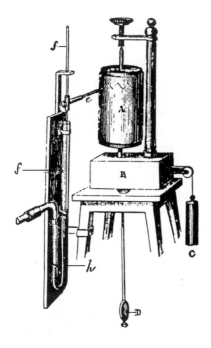

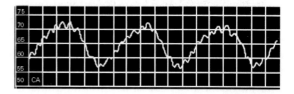

FIGURE 2. Kymographion of K.F. Ludwig (1816–1895). Blood pressure variations recorded by the Ludwig Kymographion.

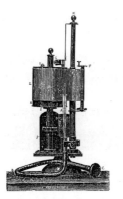

FIGURE 3. Sphygmograph of C. Ozanam (1824–1890).

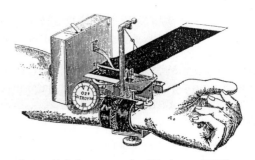

FIGURE 5. Sphygmograph of Dudgeon (1881).

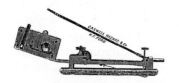

FIGURE 4. Sphygmograph of F.A. Mahomed (1849–1884).

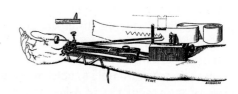

FIGURE 6. Sphygmograph of Brondel (1879).

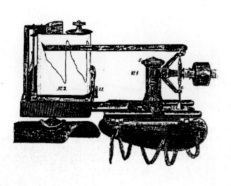

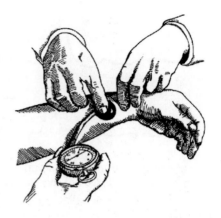

FIGURE 7. Sphygmometrograph of M.A. Philadelphien (1896).

FIGURE 8. Sphygmomanometer of P.C. Potin (1825–1901).

with increasing rigidity of the arterial wall due to arteriosclerosis. It was recognized quite early that the elasticity of an artery is related to the velocity of volume pulse waves propagated through it. Moens (1878) derived a mathematical expression for the velocity of the front of a pulse wave travelling along an artery as a function of inter alia the elasticity coefficient, the thickness of the arterial wall and the end-diastolic diameter of the lumen of the vessel. Moens also proved the validity of the formula through experiments on elastic tubing.

The velocity of transmission of the pulse wave was used as a clinical index of arterial elasticity by Bramwell and Hill in 1922, and then by a large number of authors using different methods: Bazett et al. in 1922, Beyerholm in 1922, Hickson in 1924, Sands in 1925, Turner in 1927, Hallock in 1934, Haynes in 1936, Steele in 1937, etc. The relationship between the PWV and the elastic properties of the wall in elastic tubes has been extensively studied from the theoretical and experimental points of view *(figures 9, 10)*. Despite its noninvasive nature, sensitivity and good reproducibility, determination of

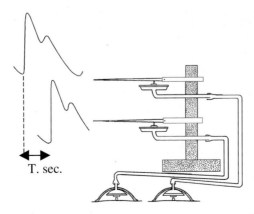

T. sec.

FIGURE 9. Two drum methods with two ideal pulse curves (1958).

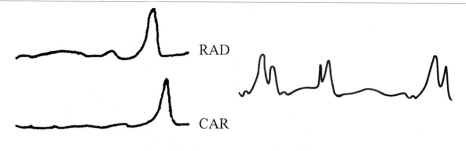

RAD

CAR

Radial (RAD) and carotid (CAR) sphygmograms recorded on separate leads.

Radial and carotid sphygmograms recorded on same lead.

FIGURE 10. PWV determination by Bramwell and Hill (1922).

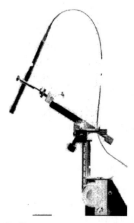

FIGURE 11. Millar® Sphygmographic tonometer (1988).

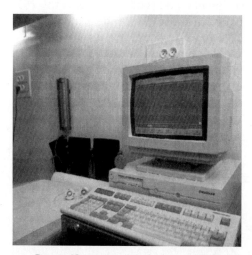

FIGURE 12. Automatic calculation of PWV. The Complior® device.

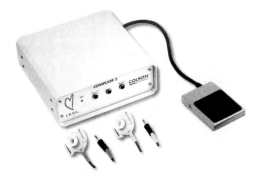

FIGURE 13. Separate modulus for PWV measurement. The Complior® II device.

PWV was not applied to clinical practice because its recording, and calculation were difficult and time-consuming. In fact, in contrast to pulse wave recording, which is simple and rapidly obtained, the manual determination of the pulse wave upstroke point inflection, the measurement of the time delay between two waves, and the calculation of the mean values are tedious and time-consuming [12, 14, 17-25]. The recent developments of noninvasive methods such as Doppler ultrasonic techniques, pressure transducers, and applanation tonometry for registration of arterial flow and pressure waves, respectively added to new principles of analysis, and automatic and computerized calculation open up a new era in the clinical applications of the analysis of the contour, amplitude and velocity of the pressure pulse *(figures 11–13)*. This book is largely directed towards the clinical application of the automatic method to determine the arterial PWV.

REFERENCES

1 Arnett DK, Evans GW, Riley WA. Arterial stiffness: a new cardiovascular risk factor? Am J Epidemiol 1994 ; 140 : 664-82.

2 Kannel WB. Blood pressure as a cardiovascular risk factor. Prevention and treatment. JAMA 1996 ; 275 : 1571-6.

3 The sixth report of the Joint National Committee on prevention, detection, evaluation, and treatment of high blood pressure. NIH Publications n° 98-4080 ; 1997.

4 McDonald DA. Blood flow in arteries: theoretical, experimental and clinical principles, 4th ed. London: Arnold; 1998. p. 77-142, p. 216-69, p. 283-359, p. 398-437.

5 O'Rourke M. Mechanical principles in arterial disease. Hypertension 1995 ; 26 : 2-9.

6 Safar ME, Frohlich ED. The arterial system in hypertension. A prospective view. Hypertension 1995 ; 26 : 10-4.

7 Asmar R, Topouchian J, Benetos A, Sayegh F, Mourad JJ, Safar M. Non-invasive evaluation of arterial abnormalities in hypertensive patients. J Hypertens 1997 ; 15 Suppl 2 : 99-107.

8 Gosse P, Guillo P, Ascher G, Clementy J. Assessment of arterial distensibility by monitoring the timing of Korotkoff sounds. Am J Hypertens 1994 ; 7 : 228-33.

9 Laurent S, Vanhoutte P, Cavero I, Chabrier PE, Dupuis B, Elghozi JL, et al. The arterial wall: a new pharmacological and therapeutic target. Fundam Clin Pharmacol 1996 ; 10 : 243-57.

10 Girerd X, Mourad JJ, Copie X, Moulin C, Acar C, Safar ME, et al. Noninvasive detection of an increased vascular mass in untreated hypertensive patients. Am J Hypertens 1994 ; 7 : 1076-84.

11 Asmar R, Benetos A, Topouchian J, Laurent P, Panier B, Brisac AM, et al. Assessment of arterial distensibility by automatic pulse wave velocity measurement. Validation and clinical application studies. Hypertension 1995 ; 26 : 485-90.

12 Bramwell JC, Hill AV. Velocity of transmission of the pulse wave and elasticity of arteries. Lancet 1922 ; 1 : 891-2.

13 Lehman ED, Parker JR, Hopkins KD, Taylor MG, Gosling RG. Validation and reproductibility of pressure-corrected aortic distensibility measurements using pulse-wave velocity Doppler ultrasound. J Biomed Engl 1993 ; 15 : 221-8.

14 Bazett HC, Dreyer NB. Measurements of pulse wave velocity. Am J Physiol 1922 ; 63 : 94-109.

15 Riva-Rocci S. Un nuovo sfigmomanometro. Gazz Med Torino 1896 ; 47 : 981-96.

16 Korotkoff NS. A contribution to the problem of methods for the determination of blood pressure. Bull Imp Military Med Acad St. Petersburg 1905 ; 11 : 365-7.

17 Moens AI. Die Pulscurve, Leiden, 1878.

18 Bramwell JC, Hill AV. The velocity of the pulse wave in man. Proc Royal Soc London 1922 ; 96 : 298-306.

19 Beyerholm O. Studies of the velocity of transmission of the pulse wave in normal individuals. Acta Med Scand 1927 ; 67 : 203-35.

20 Hickson SK, McSwiney BA. Effect of respiratory movements on pulse wave velocity. J Physiol 1924 ; 59 : 217-20.

21 Sands J. Studies in pulse wave velocity. III. pulse wave velocity in pathological conditions. Am J Physiol 1924 ; 71 : 519.

22 Turner RH, Herrmann GR. pulse wave velocity under varying conditions in normal and abnormal human cardiovascular systems. J Clin Invest 1927 ; 4 : 430.

23 Hallock P. Arterial elasticity in man in relation to age as evaluated by the pulse wave velocity method. Arch Int Med 1934 ; 54 : 770.

24 Haynes FW, Ellis LB, Weiss S. pulse wave velocity and arterial elasticity in arterial hypertension, arteriosclerosis, and related conditions. Am Heart J 1936 ; 11 : 385-401.

25 Steele JM. Interpretation of arterial elasticity from measurements of pulse wave velocities. Am Heart J 1937 ; 7 : 452-65.

II
CHAPTER

Arterial pulse wave

The arterial pulse is a fluctuation caused by heart contraction and occurs at the same frequency as the heart rate. The ejection of blood from the left ventricle through the aortic valve in the aorta leads to flow, pressure, and diameter pulsations throughout the arterial tree [1]. Many of these fluctuations can be considered as 'pulse', but usually clinicians refer to pulse only as the arterial pressure pulses which can be palpated in large accessible arteries. In order to understand the arterial hemodynamics and the three different pulsations (*figure 1*) which have been used to measure PWV, this chapter will briefly treat the flow and diameter pulses, putting more emphasis on the pressure pulse, which is at the present time the most frequently used method for measuring PWV.

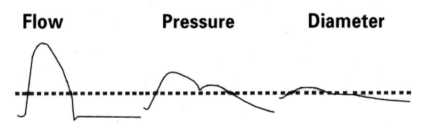

Flow   **Pressure**   **Diameter**

FIGURE 1. Fluctuations in amplitude of flow, pressure, and diameter in a large artery. The pulsatile flow fluctuation in a large artery is $\simeq$ 300% of the mean flow, considerably more than the pulsatile pressure fluctuation, which is around 60% of the mean pressure, and the tiny fluctuation in diameter which is less than 10%.

PRESSURE WAVE

The contraction of the left ventricular myocardium and the ejection of blood into the ascending aorta generates a pressure wave which will travel along the arterial wall throughout the body. Because of its amplification, the amplitude of the pressure fluctuation in the peripheral arteries is usually greater than in the large arteries close to the heart [2, 3].

FLOW WAVE

The ejection of blood from the heart into the aorta generates a pulsatile blood flow which can usually be evaluated by Doppler. This ultrasonic technique measures the velocity of the blood pumped into the arteries. Because of the cushioning properties of the arterial wall and the increase in the cross-sectional area of the arteries, the amplitude of the flow fluctuation is usually greater in the large than in the peripheral arteries [4].

DIAMETER WAVE

Modification of the distension pressure within the artery causes an identical modification of the arterial diameter. However, the relationship between diameter and pressure is curvilinear because of the nonlinear elastic properties of the arterial wall. Moreover, these properties differ from one artery to the other, according to their structure. In fact, for the same modification of the distension pressure, the large elastic arteries will present a greater modification of their diameter than the small muscular arteries [1-3]. The amplitude of the diameter fluctuation is usually very small, and its evaluation is difficult and needs to be assessed using sophisticated methods.

PROPERTIES OF THE PRESSURE WAVE

Pulse pressure can be recorded invasively by catheter or noninvasively by an external pressure transducer. Several noninvasive methods have been used for pulse recording: sphygmograph, external volume capsule, plethysmography, piezoelectric transducer, tonometer, etc., each having some specific limits and advantages. Because the pressure pulse waveform changes in both amplitude and contour as it travels from the aorta to the peripheral arteries, the advantage of the noninvasive pressure transducer is its ability to record pulse waves in different arterial sites [5-7].

In order to understand arterial pulsation, which is dependent on ventricular contraction and the properties of the arterial and arteriolar systems, it is necessary to consider arterial hemodynamics and the concept of wave travel and reflection, which determine the relationship between systolic and diastolic pressures in central and peripheral arteries. In fact, it is well established that the pulse pressure wave must be analyzed as a superposition of two (and sometimes three) separate waves: the incident wave traveling from the heart to the periphery, and the reflected wave traveling from the periphery and the site of wave reflection to the heart [2-3] *(figure 2)*.

The incident wave depends on the left ventricular ejection and the arterial stiffness (PWV), whereas the reflected wave is related to arterial stiffness and the potential sites of wave reflection.

In young adults, where arteries are distensible and thus the wave travel velocity relatively low, the reflected wave is seen only in diastole. In older subjects, where the arteries are less distensible and thus the pulse wave travel velocity high, the reflected wave is seen in the rising limb of the systolic pressure wave with a substantial superposition

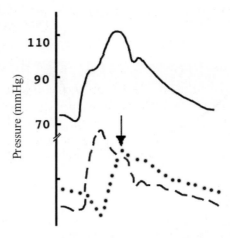

FIGURE 2. Breakdown of the measured pulse pressure (—) into a forward incident wave (– – –) and a backward reflected wave (••••).

of the two waves, causing an increase in systolic blood pressure. This characteristic change in shape of the pulse wave with age is attributed to an increase in aortic stiffness and PWV, with earlier return of reflected waves from peripheral sites *(figures 3, 4)*. Thus, the amplitude and the contour of the pressure and the flow waves in systemic arteries can be explained on the basis of the arterial hemodynamics, stiffness, and wave reflection [8-10].

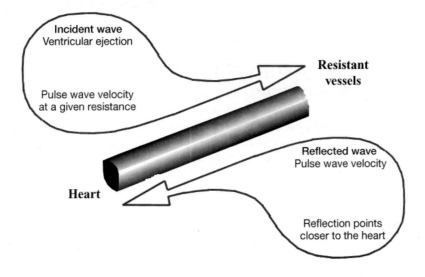

FIGURE 3. Determinants of the arterial pulse pressure.

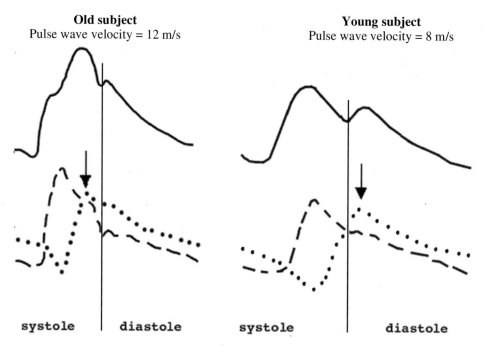

FIGURE 4. Pressure waves in young and old subjects.
Measured wave (—); backward wave (••••); forward wave (– – –).

RELATIONSHIP BETWEEN PRESSURE AND FLOW WAVES

The relationship between pressure and flow in an artery can be described as the vascular impedance. Impedance is determined by the properties of the arterial tree beyond the point of measurement.

The comparison of pressure behaviour and flow waves in arteries showed that mean pressure falls slightly, that pressure variations increase, and that flow pulsations diminish as they travel from the heart to the periphery *(figure 5)*.

CHANGES OF PRESSURE PULSE WAVE WITH AGE IN DIFFERENT ARTERIES

From the heart to the peripheral arteries, the pressure pulse shows a progressive change in amplitude and contour. In fact, mean blood pressure decreases slightly, whereas pulse pressure increases substantially due to an increase in systolic blood pressure and to a smaller decrease in diastolic blood pressure. This increase in the systolic blood pressure in the peripheral arteries is mainly related to an earlier reflected wave which arrives during systole and not diastole, because of the shortened distance to the peripheral reflection site *(figure 5)*.

• In the aorta, ejection of blood dilates the aortic wall and generates a pressure wave. In young adults, this pulse presents a rounded top and a second wave after the incisura which marks aortic valve closure. The second wave is related to the peripheral reflection, principally from the lower part of the body.

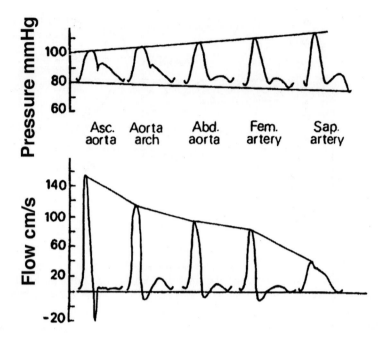

FIGURE 5. Changes in the contour and amplitude of the pressure and flow waves in arteries as they travel from the heart to the periphery. (Adapted with permission from: Mc Donald DA. Blood flow in arteries: theoretical, experimental and clinical principles. 3rd ed. London: E. Arnold; 1960.)

• In the lower limb, the pulse pressure rises progressively between the aorta and the lower limb. The peak systolic pressure increases and a secondary wave is apparent. This increase in systolic blood pressure is attributed to the summation of the incident wave and the reflected wave, since both are close to the peripheral reflecting sites. The secondary diastolic wave in lower body arteries is due to the reflected wave from the upper to the lower body.

• In the upper limb, the peak systolic pressure is greater than in the aorta. Normally, the pulse presents an early systolic peak, followed by a late systolic shoulder before the dicrotic notch and another wave immediately thereafter. The early peak is due to the initial pressure impulse; the late systolic shoulder and early diastolic wave are due to wave reflection from the lower body.

The mechanisms of the changes in the contour and amplitude of the pressure wave can be explained by considering the 'pressure transfer function'. This amplification is related to the intensity of wave reflection, to the difference in stiffness between central and distal arteries, the blood pressure level and, as would be expected, PWV [2, 3, 5-10].

With increasing age, hypertension, and arterio- and atherosclerosis, the arterial wall thickness increases and presents functional and structural abnormalities. These alterations predominate much more in the central elastic arteries than in the distal arteries, and thus generate an increase in central pressure pulse *(figures 6, 7)* [11-17]. In fact, with

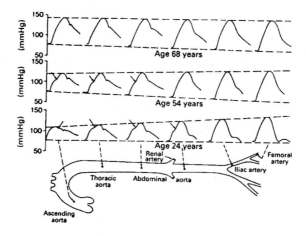

FIGURE 6. Pressure wave recorded in different sites in three adult subjects. In the oldest subject, there is little amplification; however, in the youngest, the amplitude increases by ≃ 60%. (Adapted with permission from: O'Rourke MF, Safar M, Dzau VJ. Arterial vasodilation. London: E. Arnold; 1993.)

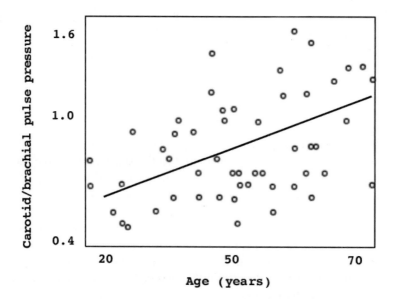

FIGURE 7. Relationship between the ratio of carotid/brachial pulse pressure and age ($r = 0.52$; $p < 0.001$). The amplification of the pressure wave between carotid and brachial artery decreases with age.

increasing age and arterial stiffening, the modifications in the contour and amplitude of the aortic pressure pulse are associated with a decrease in the pulse amplification between central and peripheral arteries. Therefore, in young adults, the distal arterial pulse is around 50% higher than that in the aorta, whereas in the older subjects, it is almost identical.

REFERENCES

1 McDonald DA. Blood flow in arteries: theorical, experimental and clinical principles, 4th ed. London: Arnold; 1998. p. 77-142, p. 216-69, p. 283-359, p. 398-437.

2 O'Rourke MF, Kelly R, Avolio A. The arterial pulse. Philadelphia - London: Lea & Febiger; 1992.

3 Safar M. Arteries in clinical hypertension. New York: Lippincott-Raven. 1996. p. 21-30.

4 Lehmann ED, Hopkins KD, Gosling RG. Aortic compliance measurements using Doppler ultrasound: in vivo biochemical correlates. Ultrasound Med Biol 1993 ; 19 : 683-710.

5 Kelly R, Daley J, Avolio A, O'Rourke M. Arterial dilation and reduced wave reflection. Hypertension 1989 ; 14 : 14-21.

6 Kelly R, Hayward C, Avolio A, O'Rourke M. Noninvasive determination of age-related changes in the human arterial pulse. Circulation 1989 ; 80 : 1652-9.

7 London GM. Large artery function and alterations in hypertension. J Hypertens 1995 ; 13 Suppl 2 : 35-8.

8 Latham RD. Pulse propagation in the systemic arterial tree. In: Westerhof N, Gross DR, eds. Vascular dynamics: physiological perspectives. New York and London: Plenum Press; 1989. p. 49-68.

9 London GM, Guérin AP, Pannier B, Marchais SJ, Métivier F, Safar ME. Arterial wave reflections and increased systolic and pulse pressure in chronic uremia. Study using noninvasive carotid pulse waveform registration. Hypertension 1992 ; 20 : 10-9.

10 Taylor MG. Wave travel in arteries and the design of the cardiovascular system. In: Attinger EO, ed. Pulsatile blood flow. New York: McGraw Hill; 1964. p. 343-7.

11 Asmar R, Benetos A, London GM, Hugue C, Weiss Y, Topouchian J, et al. Aortic distensibility in normotensive, untreated and treated hypertensive patients. Blood Pressure 1995 ; 4 : 48-54.

12 Boutouyrie P, Laurent S, Girerd X, Benetos A, Lacolley P, Abergel E, et al. Common carotid artery stiffness and patterns of left ventricular hypertrophy in hypertensive patients. Hypertension 1995 ; 25 : 651-9.

13 Draaijer P, Kool MJ, Maessen JM, Van Bortel LM, de Leeuw PW, Van Hoof JP, et al. Vascular distensibility. J Hypertens 1993; 11: 1199-207.

14 Laurent S. Arterial wall hypertrophy and stiffness in essential hypertensive patients. Hypertension 1995 ; 26 : 355-62.

15 O'Rourke MF, Kelly RP. Wave reflection in the systemic circulation and its implications in ventricular function. J Hypertens 1993 ; 11 : 327-37.

16 Safar ME, Frohlich ED. The arterial system in hypertension. A prospective view. Hypertension 1995 ; 26 : 10-4.

17 Benetos A, Laurent S, Hoeks AP, Boutouyrie PH, Safar ME. Arterial alterations with ageing and high blood pressure: a non-invasive study of carotid and femoral arteries. Arterioscler Thromb 1993 ; 13 : 90-7.

III

CHAPTER

Pulse wave velocity
Principles and measurement

Large-artery damage is the major contributor to cardiovascular disease, which represents the leading cause of mortality and morbidity in industrialized countries. This high incidence emphasizes the importance of early evaluation of the arterial abnormalities which constitute the common lesion of major organ damages due to cardiovascular risk factors. Several methods can be used to analyse the structure and function of the large arteries. Most of these are complex or need sophisticated technical equipment, which limits their application in clinical practice [1-5]. Among the noninvasive and simple methods of evaluating arteries, PWV measurement is widely used as an index of arterial elasticity and stiffness. This method is simple, accurate and repro-ducible, and thus can easily be applied in clinical evaluation and trials [6-10].

DEFINITION

The contraction of the left ventricular myocardium and ejection of blood into the ascending aorta dilate the aortic wall and generate a pulse wave, which is propagated throughout the arterial tree at a finite speed. This propagation velocity constitutes an index of arterial distensibility and stiffness. Higher velocity corresponds to higher arterial rigidity, and thus to lower distensibility *(figure 1)*.

PRINCIPLES

Arterial pulse can be analysed on the basis of different pulsations: the flow waves, the diameter waves and the pressure waves. In order to facilitate the comprehension of the PWV principles, we will consider hereafter only the arterial pressure pulse.

The pressure pulse generated by ventricular ejection is propagated throughout the arterial tree at a speed determined by the elastic and geometric properties of the arterial wall and the characteristics (density) of the contained fluid (blood). Since blood is an incompressible fluid and is contained in elastic conduits (arteries), the energy propaga-

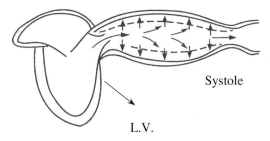

Systole

L.V.

FIGURE 1. PWV. LVE generates a pulse wave which will propagate throughout the arterial wall at a finite speed. Propagation velocity is determined by the elastic and geometric properties of the arterial wall, and the characteristics of the fluid (blood density). Higher velocity = higher stiffness.

tion occurs predominantly along the walls of the arteries and not through the incompressible blood. The properties of the arterial wall, its thickness, and the arterial lumen are thus the major factors of PWV. The use of PWV as an index of arterial elasticity and stiffness, as determined from the time delay between the foot of pulse pressure waves recorded at two different sites and the distance between those recording sites, has been extensively analysed. In fact, it has been well established that PWV in an elastic tube is related to the elastic properties of the wall. This has been analysed from the theoretical and experimental points of view in a number of studies performed on fluid-filled tubes, excised segments of arteries and in intact human subjects. The relationships between PWV, pressure, tension, distensibility, and tube volume have been made by Bramwell, Downing, and Hill on segments of excised carotid artery, and by Hamilton, Remington, and Dow on mercury-filled Gooch tubing and on cadaver aortas. These physical concepts have been formalised in many mathematical models, where the arterial segment has been considered as a thin-walled tube (by Womersley) or as a thick-walled viscoelastic tube (by Cox) [11-23]. The study of models, taking into account the main features of the human arterial tree, confirmed that the PWV given by the well-known Moens-Korteweg equation or the Bramwell-Hill equation presents a good approximation and evaluation.

$$\text{Moens-Korteweg equation: } PWV^2 = E.h \,/\, 2r.\rho$$

where h is the arterial wall thickness, r is the internal radius, ρ is blood density, and E is the Young modulus of the wall. $E = \Delta P.D \,/h.\Delta D$, where ΔP and ΔD are changes in pressure and diameter, and h is the wall thickness. The Young modulus represents the ratio (or the slope) of the stress/strain relationship. It reflects the arterial wall properties *(figure 2)*.

The assumptions underlying the Moens-Korteweg equation were explored in 1960 by Bergel [23], who suggests a corrected equation taking into consideration the Poisson ratio (σ), which is the ratio of transverse to longitudinal strain. This ratio is a characteristic property of the material. The value of σ for the arterial wall is close to 0.5. $PWV^2 = E.h \,/\, 2r.\rho \,(1-\sigma^2)$

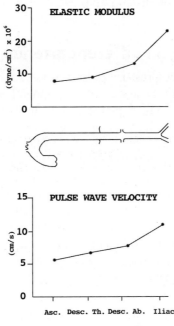

FIGURE 2. Elastic modulus and PWV in different arterial sites.
Both increase as the distance from the heart increases. (Adapted from Nichols et al. [24].)

Bramwell-Hill equation: $PWV^2 = \Delta P.V / \Delta V.\rho$

where ΔP and ΔV are the changes in pressure and volume, V is the baseline volume, and ρ is blood density. Since volume distensibility = $\Delta V/\Delta P.V$, it can be calculated from the PWV using a modification of the Bramwell-Hill equation, that distensibility = $D = 1 / \rho (PWV)^2$.

It can also be expressed as compliance by unit length, and the equation becomes: Compliance = $\pi.R^2/ \rho.(PWV)^2$, where R is the arterial radius and ρ is the blood viscosity.

Pulse wave velocity and impedance

Another commonly used measure of arterial stiffness is the aortic characteristic impedance (Zc), which can be determined from pressure and flow waves recorded simultaneously in the ascending aorta by relating the corresponding frequency components of pressure and flow waves in that artery.

The term impedance should be used when considering pulsatile flow and pressure in arteries, and the term resistance should be confined to the steady or mean flow (not pulsatile). Vascular impedance describes the relationship between pressure and flow. The characteristic impedance (Zc) is defined as the ratio of oscillatory pressure to flow at the input of a tube in which no reflected wave returns to the origin; it is usually estimated by averaging values of the modulus at high frequencies. When expressed in terms of linear flow velocity (dyne.s.cm^{-3}, not volume flow), characteristic impedance is numerically very similar to PWV according to the Water-Hammer formula: $PWV = Zc.\rho$, where Zc is characteristic impedance, PWV = PWV, and ρ = blood viscosity. Both

PWV and Zc are dependent on distending pressure in a non linear fashion over a wide pressure range [25-27].

Pulse wave velocity in different arteries

As mentioned previously, the pressure pulse shows progressive changes in amplitude and contour as it travels from the aorta to the peripheral arteries. This amplification or 'pressure transfer function' can be explained on the basis of the arterial hemodynamics, stiffness and wave reflection. It leads to an increase in systolic and pulse pressure in the peripheral arteries. With increasing age, the arterial alterations are predominant mainly in the central elastic arteries, and therefore the pulse amplification between central and peripheral arteries decreases with ageing and atherosclerosis. Elsewhere, according to the Bramwell – Hill and Moens – Korteweg equations, the propagation velocity of the pulse wave along the arterial wall is related to the distension blood pressure, blood density, arterial diameter, and the thickness and elastic properties of the arterial wall. Several studies have shown that PWV increases from the aorta to the periphery *(figure 3)*. This increase in PWV may be considered as resulting from several factors (see also the chapter on determinants of PWV).

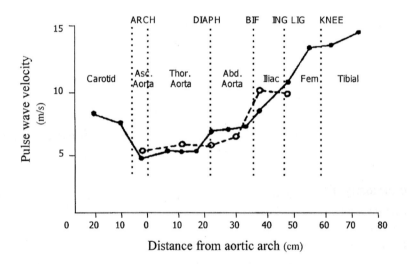

FIGURE 3. Progressive increase in PWV with increasing distance from the heart in animals (——) and humans (-----). (Adapted from McDonald [28] and Latham et al. [29].)

Blood pressure

PWV is related to blood pressure; since pulse pressure increases as it travels from the aorta to the periphery, PWV increases throughout the arterial tree.

Arterial diameter and wall thickness

The overall pattern of the arterial network and its branches was considered in detail by Hess in 1927 [30]. Different techniques have been used to measure the arterial diameter in different conditions (in situ, in vivo, in animal, in human, postmortem, etc.). It is well known that the diameter or radius and the cross-sectional area of the arteries decrease from the ascending aorta to the periphery *(figure 4)*. It is well established that the thickness/diameter ratio, which represents the relative wall thickness, increases in large arteries with increasing distance from the heart, mainly in older subjects *(figure 5)*.

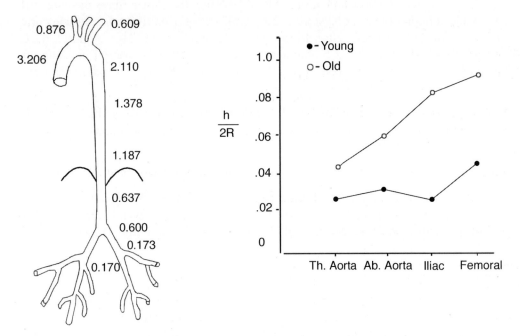

FIGURE 4. Mean internal cross-sectional area (cm²) at various sites in the aorta and its main branches. (Adapted from Patel et al. [31].)

FIGURE 5. Relative wall thickness (h = wall thickness; R = radius) of different arterial sites in young and older subjects. (Adapted from Learoyd and Taylor [32].)

Blood viscosity, density

It has been described that in small tubes, the apparent viscosity at higher rates of shear is smaller than in large tubes. This progressive diminution with tube size begins to be detectable in tubes whose internal diameter is less than 1 mm. The viscoelastic properties of red cells change with age as well; at constant shear stress, young cells deform more than old ones. Except in some cardiovascular diseases where blood density may play an important role, usually in clinical practice, it is considered equal in the vascular bed and evaluated using a hematocrit [19-23, 33-37].

Elastic properties of the arterial wall

The elastic modulus of the arterial wall represents the ratio between stress/strain and reflects its properties. The histologic structure of the arterial wall has been described in detail [38]. The predominant elastic materials of the arterial wall are collagen and elastin; another major constituent is the smooth muscle, which cannot properly be considered a true elastic material but contributes to the wall tension. The distribution of elastin and collagen differs strikingly between the central and peripheral arteries. In the proximal aorta, elastin is the dominant component, while in the distal aorta, the reverse is true. In peripheral arteries, collagen and smooth muscle cells dominate. The elastic modulus of collagen is much higher than that of elastin, so that as the distance from the heart increases, the arteries become stiffer, and the elastic modulus and PWV increase *(figure 2)*. This relation can be easily verified by the Moens-Korteweg equation. Elsewhere, it is important to note that at low and normal blood pressure, the elastin fibres mediate stiffness, while at higher pressure (systolic > 200 mmHg), collagen fibres do, allowing arterial expansion but also protection from wall yield and rupture. This biphasic elastic content of the artery produces a nonlinear relationship between arterial pressure and diameter. The smooth muscle contributes to the stiffness of the arterial wall by the transfer of tension from one type of fibre to the other.

All these elements clearly justify the nonuniform arterial elasticity in the arterial tree; the difference in distensibility of the aorta and peripheral arteries is made manifest as different values of PWV.

Ageing

Age, arteriosclerosis and atherosclerosis affect the arterial tree differently. In fact, the alterations predominate much more in the central elastic arteries than in the distal arteries and thus will modify the central and peripheral PWV differently. The effect of age on PWV will be treated in detail in chapter IV.

Relation between aortic and brachial pulse wave velocity

Using a simple transmission line model, values of PWV in the aorta and the brachial artery can be used to estimate the amplification of the pressure pulse due to nonuniform arterial elasticity. From the Water-Hammer formula, PWV is related to the characteristic impedance (Zc, impedance in the absence of wave reflection) of an artery and to blood density (ρ) as follows:

$$PWV = Zc.\rho.$$

In this model, in the absence of wave reflection, the ratio of proximal (p) to distal (d) pressure amplitude (P) is proportional to the square root of the characteristic impedance:

$$Pp/Pd = \sqrt{\frac{Zc\ proximal}{Zc\ distal}}$$

If we replace impedance (Zc) by PWV, the equation becomes:

$$Brachial\ pulse\ pressure\ /\ Aortic\ pulse\ pressure = \sqrt{\frac{Brachial\ PWV}{Aortic\ PWV}}$$

Thus, the ratio between brachial and aortic pulse wave velocities may be used as an index to estimate the amplification of the pulse due to nonuniform arterial elasticity.

This is important to note here, because of peripheral wave reflection and pulse wave amplification that this calculation is an underestimation of the true value since it is based only on one mechanism of nonuniform elasticity and does not consider the effect of ejection time, which has been shown to be a significant factor. When this limitation is taken into account, the method does at least provide a means of estimating the minimum difference between aortic and brachial artery pulse pressure *(figure 6)*.

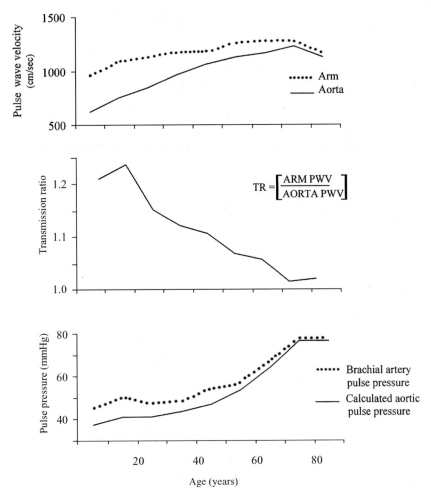

FIGURE 6. Relations between age/aortic and arm PWV. (Adapted from Avolio et al. [40].)
Transmission ratio (TR) calculated as arm PWV/aorta PWV. Measured brachial artery
pulse pressure (BPP) in the same subjects and calculated aortic pulse pressure (APP): APP = BPP/TR.

Even if several authors considered this approach, few studies have been performed to evaluate the ratio between pulse wave velocities as a marker of pressure wave amplitude changes or an index to estimate the amplification of the pulse due to nonuniform arterial elasticity. From this viewpoint, Pannier et al. [39] analysed the ratio between the arm (brachial-radial) and the aortic (carotid-femoral) pulse wave velocities in normotensive and hypertensive patients of the same age. Their results showed similar ratios in normotensives and hypertensives, decreasing with age to the same extent in both populations; the ratio was independent of the blood pressure level and was influenced only by age. The authors suggested the use of the PWV ratio as a marker of the arterial system, which is independent of the blood pressure level in hypertensives, and influenced to a considerable extent by age; this marker indicates the changes in pressure wave transmission along the arterial tree (*figure 7*).

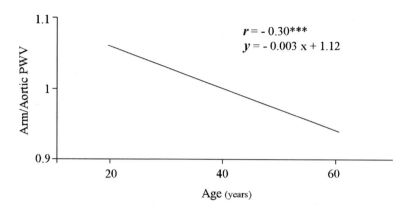

$r = - 0.30***$
$y = - 0.003 \, x + 1.12$

FIGURE 7. Relationship between age and the ratio of the arm/aortic pulse wave velocities.
(Adapted from Pannier et al. [39].)

TABLE I. Values of arterial pulse wave velocities measured in different arteries.

Artery	PWV m/s Mean value (range)	Reference
Ascending aorta	5.20	Luchsinger et al. (1964) [41]
	5.45	Merillon et al. (1980) [42]
	6.68	Murgo et al. (1980) [27]
	4.40	Latham et al. (1985) [43]
Thoracic aorta	4.00	Luchsinger et al. (1964) [41]
	5.30	Latham et al. (1985) [43]
	(5.50 – 6.50)	Wezler et al. (1939) [44]
	5.80	Learoyd et al. (1966) [32]
Abdominal aorta	5.00	Luchsinger et al. (1964) [41]
	5.70	Latham et al. (1985) [43]
	(5.50 – 6.20)	Learoyd et al. (1966) [32]
Iliac artery	8.80	Latham et al. (1985) [43]
Femoral artery	8.00	Kapal et al. (1951) [45]
	9.70	Zangeneh et al. (1967) [46]
Carotid artery	6.80 – 8.30	Bramwell et al. (1922) [12]
Radial artery	4.90	Sands et al. (1925) [47]
Pulmonary artery	1.68	Milnor et al. (1969) [48]
	1.82	Caro et al. (1962) [49]

CALCULATION OF PULSE WAVE VELOCITY

The pulse wave generated by the left ventricular myocardium contraction and blood ejection is propagated throughout the arterial tree at a speed determined by the elastic and geometric properties of the arterial wall and the blood density. This velocity is calculated using the formula: Velocity = D/T, where D represents the distance traveled by the pulse between two recording sites, the proximal and distal, and T represents the transit time needed by the front wave to travel from one site to the other; it is determined by the time delay between the two corresponding recorded front waves *(figure 8)*. As mentioned in the previous chapter, this propagation velocity constitutes a well-established distensibility index of the arterial wall; it is derived by a calculation from two measured parameters: the distance and the time delay. Considering that respiration modifies the intrathoracic pressure, the vessel wall tensions and therefore the arterial blood pressure, PWV varies with respiratory variability. For this reason, the considered value of PWV usually represents the mean value calculated on the basis of about ten consecutive recorded beats to cover a complete respiratory cycle. The purpose of this chapter is to describe the different methods of: 1) recording pulse wave signals; 2) measuring the covered distance; 3) determining the wave 'foot' or the 'characteristic' point of the wave; and 4) calculating the time delay between the proximal and distal waves.

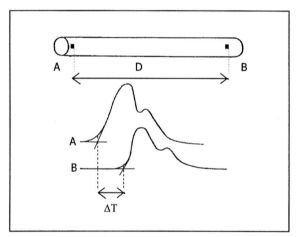

FIGURE 8. PWV measurement.
A = wave recorded by the proximal transducer. B = wave recorded by the distal transducer.
ΔT = time delay between the foot waves. D = distance traveled by the wave.

Recordings of pulse signals

Which pulse signals?

As mentioned in chapter II, arterial pulse wave is related to three different pulsations: flow, pressure, and diameter fluctuations. These arterial pulses may be detected and displayed as time-varying signals and thus used for determining PWV. The time delay measured between the foot of proximal and distal waves of any of these three signals is almost identical. Schematically, the techniques for measuring these signals can be divided into invasive and noninvasive methods: the latter are atraumatic and have the advantages of being able to record the pulse wave in different peripheral arterial sites and to be repeated in the same patient. These will be described in detail, whereas the former will just be mentioned briefly.

■ Pressure–volume pulse waves

The pressure pulse can be measured invasively using intra-arterial pressure-sensitive high-fidelity transducers. This technique is usually reserved for catheterization diagnosis, intraoperative and critical care monitoring, and for some specific research applications. Two different techniques have been primarily used: a catheter with an external pressure transducer and a catheter-mounted transducer.

For noninvasive measurements, pressure-sensitive transducers can be used, but their application is restricted to superficial arteries where the pulse can be palpated. External pulse recording usually employs air- or fluid-containing capsules placed over pulse points. The volume/pressure pulsations of an artery are transmitted in the radial direction and are then detected by the capsules and magnified by the displacement of air or fluid. These recorded pulsations differ from the pressure signal detected at the arterial wall, since displacement in the radial direction is not directly proportional to the changes in intra-arterial pressure. Moreover, some precautions must be taken when this method is used: the choice of a large volume capsule may induce artefacts from adjacent venous pulsations, and the hold-down force applied to maintain the capsule may modify the wave forms. The pressure-sensitive transducer should have a large frequency bandwidth (for example, 0.1–100 Hz) to cover the principal frequency harmonics of the pressure wave at different heart rates and thus allows its application for PWV measurement in a clinical setting [50].

Another pressure/volume pulse recording method has been widely employed using plethysmography. This method measures the volume variations using a mercury-filled silastic tube (mercury plethysmography) or a light source and a photo-detector (photo-plethysmography). Like the previous pressure/volume transducer, this technique is limited by the assumption of linearity between pressure and volume changes [34]. Recently, the application of tonometer principles, described by Mackay et al. in 1960 for intra-ocular pressure measurement, to peripheral arterial pressure measurement, allowed the development of the Millar sphygmographic tonometer (1988). This technique employs a pencil-shaped probe incorporating a Millar micromanometer in its tip. Since it is well known that applanation of a pressure-containing structure curved surface under the pressure sensor allows direct measurement of the pressure within the structure, this device allows pressure wave shape recording as well as arterial pressure measurement [51, 52].

■ Flow waves

Left ventricular myocardium contraction and blood ejection into the aorta generate a pulsatile blood flow. The blood propagation velocity is usually measured by a noninvasive ultrasound technique, transcutaneous Doppler transducers. This method can detect the flow velocity pulse in the superficial peripheral arteries and also in other, less externally palpable arteries, such as the aorta. Thus, for some authors, the use of this method is more suitable than the use of pressure/volume wave recording, since it is not restricted to palpable arteries. This latter point must be considered carefully because, like all other methods, the Doppler signal and its quality are dependent on observer experience, and since it is directly related to the probe application angle it may represent a large inter-observer variability [8, 53, 54]. For PWV measurement, the Doppler technique used is usually continuous Doppler, using high-frequency ultrasound (8 or 10 MHz) for the superficial arteries and low-frequency ultrasound (2 or 4 MHz) for deeper arteries.

■ Diameter waves

As mentioned in the previous chapter, the amplitude of the diameter fluctuation is small by comparison to those of the pressure and flow waves, and its measurement should be performed using a sophisticated method based on ultrasound technique and the 'Echo-Tracking' system. Recently, Benthin et al. [68] described a specific ultrasonic instru-ment to calculate PWV using a two-dimensional real-time, B-mode image, with a com-puter-controlled digital analysis. The use of such sophisticated and complex methods may considerably limit PWV application measurement in clinical settings, particularly in large trials [3, 55].

Recording of the signals

The proximal and distal waves recorded in two different sites on the arterial tree may be collected sequentially from one site and then the other, or simultaneously from the two sites. The latter is more accurate since it records the real traveling velocity of the same wave; the former needs a fixed signal (e.g., ECG signal) and the traveling velocity is cal-culated from different waves.

The waves are usually recorded on two different leads of a paper recorder at high speed, over 100 mm/s. This high-speed paper recording is an important factor to con-sider since it influences the facility, and thus the error, of measuring the time delay between the foot of the two curves. In fact, when the two measurement sites are sepa-rated by a relatively large distance, e.g., for the aortic PWV, a paper recording speed of 100 mm/s may be sufficient, whereas when the two sites are closer, e.g., for the brachial-radial PWV, the foot of the corresponding curves are close to one other and a higher paper recording speed of 150 mm/s is recommended to facilitate the measurement of the time delay between them.

■ Successive recordings

This method is usually used when only one transducer or probe is available to detect the wave signal. The observer operates in two stages: firstly, he or she records simultaneously on a two-lead paper recorder a fixed signal, e.g., ECG, and the flow or pressure waves col-lected from one site, e.g., the proximal site. Secondly, he or she records the fixed signal and the flow or pressure wave collected from the other site, e.g., the distal site (figure 9). The time delay between the foot of the wave recorded in the proximal and the distal sites is measured indirectly by subtraction of the two time intervals $\Delta T = T2 - T1$, where T2 is the time interval measured between the fixed signal and the distal wave foot, and T1 the time interval measured between the fixed signal and the proximal wave foot. Each time interval, T1 and T2, is usually calculated on the basis of ten consecutive heartbeats.

This method is usually used when simultaneous recording of the two waves, proximal and distal, is not available. It has the disadvantage of doubling the manipulation, duration of the exam, and calculation. Elsewhere, PWV measurement according to this method is based on the traveling speed of different waves generated by different heart-beats and not on the same wave generated by the same heartbeat, as it can be performed

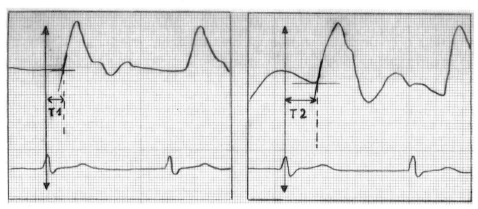

A = Recording of the proximal wave   B = Recording of the distal wave

FIGURE 9. Measurement of the time delay from successive recordings of the proximal (A)
and the distal (B) waves. The time delay between the foot of the two waves is ΔT = T2 - T1,
where T1 is the time interval measured between the ECG signal and the foot of the proximal wave
and T2 the time interval measured between the ECG signal and the foot of the distal wave.

using simultaneous recordings of the proximal and distal waves. Moreover, this method
does not consider the variability between the recordings of the proximal and the distal
sites.

■ Simultaneous recordings

This method is the most widely employed. The operator records simultaneously on a
two-lead paper recorder at high speed (100–150 mm/s) the proximal and the distal waves
collected respectively from the corresponding transducers fixed on two different sites of
the arterial tree. The main advantage of this method, which uses two transducers, is the
measurement of the real velocity of the same wave as it travels through a definite distance from one site to another *(figure 10)*. The time delay between the foot of the two
curves can be directly measured on the paper recordings. Like the previous method, the
time delay value is usually measured on the basis of ten successive heartbeats in order
to cover the variability over a complete respiratory cycle.

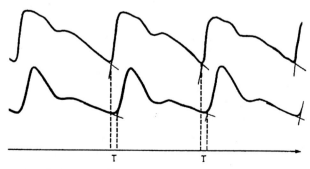

FIGURE 10. Measurement of the time delay from simultaneous recordings of the proximal (upper lead)
and the distal (lower lead) waves. The time interval (T) between the foot of the two waves is directly
measured on the paper recording.

Determination of the traveled distance

The propagation of the pulse wave is calculated according to the formula velocity = distance/time. The distance is the distance traveled between the two recordings points, the proximal and the distal; the time is the transit time needed by the wave to travel between the two sites. If the transit time measurement is critical because of the difficulties of determining the wave's characteristic points (see below), the measurement of the covered distance also has to be considered with caution. In fact, the traveled distance is directly involved in the calculated velocity value; in this regard, several of its aspects have to be considered.

Measurements of the covered distance

The covered distance between the two transducers used for pulse recordings is usually determined at the end of the examination by superficial measurement (over the skin) of the direct distance between the two middle transducers' skin traces, using a tape measure. This noninvasive, superficial measurement allows only an estimate of the covered distance; accurate measurements of the distance are obtained only with such invasive procedures as catheterization or angiography. According to the arterial territory, the recording sites, the arterial segment covered by the pulse propagation, and other parameters related to the patient's characteristics (age, weight, etc.), some critical observations on the noninvasive superficial measurements must be considered.

■ First: the arterial path length according to the propagation directions

• The two recording transducers may be placed at two sites on the same arterial axis or branch where the proximal and distal pulse waves (or blood circulation) propagate in the same direction, such as for PWV measured in the subclavian-radial, axillary-radial, brachial-radial, or femoral-tibial arterial territories, among others. In these cases, the covered distance may be estimated by direct superficial measurement, as mentioned above, with acceptable accuracy.

• The proximal and distal pulse waves may be recorded from two different arterial axis sites, where pulse waves propagate in opposite directions, such as for carotid-femoral PWV measurement. In fact, the pulse wave generated by the left ventricle contraction is propagated throughout the aorta, iliac and femoral arteries in the opposite direction than through the carotid artery. In this case, evaluating the covered distance by superficial measurement, as mentioned above, presents some margin of error; several methods and corrections have therefore been proposed:

– in order to limit the distance travelled by the pulse wave in opposite directions, some authors suggested recording the carotid wave at the common carotid artery, at the base of the neck as near as possible to the suprasternal notch, thus close to the aortic arch. Application of such a method is limited because of the difficulties in recording an ideal-quality pulse signal at this site for morphological and anatomical reasons, principally when a mechanical transducer is used for pressure wave recording [56];

– some authors suggested recording blood flow velocity with a continuous-wave Doppler ultrasound transducer placed in the left supraclavicular fossa and pointing medially to the insonate aorta close to the origin of the left subclavian artery [54]. Other authors suggested placing the Doppler probe in the suprasternal notch fossa pointing medially and left in order to record the aortic flow. Under these conditions, they suggested estimating the traveled distance by superficial measurement between the sternal notch (proximal site) and the distal site (abdominal aorta or femoral artery). There is only a limited application of such methods because of the technique of using a continuous-wave Doppler ultrasound transducer, which is highly operator-dependent [57];

– elsewhere, some authors recommended subtracting the distance between the sternal notch to the carotid location (when the common carotid is recorded at its distal part) from the total distance (e.g., carotid-femoral), because the pulse is traveling in the opposite direction. It must be noticed here that the use of such a method involves two superficial distance measurements (between the carotid site to the suprasternal notch, and the total distance), thus increasing twofold the margin of error and the bias of such measurements [14-16, 54-56, 58];

– most authors estimate the covered distance from superficial measurement of the distance between the two transducers, one positioned at the base of the neck for the right common carotid artery and the other over the right femoral artery. Several arguments have been raised to support this method: 1) not subtracting the distance traveled in the opposite direction, in order to avoid increasing errors related to supplementary distance measurement and its bias; 2) the error related to such measurement is of similar magnitude in all subjects, and thus affects only the absolute values of distance or PWV; 3) most of the studies including repeated measurements of PWV and analysis primarily consider its charge values; such admitted error, therefore, does not affect the results; and 4) because arteries become longer and more twisted with age, the path lengths determined from superficial linear measurements are generally underestimated; such underestimation may thus be balanced by not subtracting the opposite direction distance. Nevertheless, it must be noted here that applying such a method overestimates the effective pathway and hence PWV.

■ Second: the arterial path length according to the patient's clinical characteristics

Several clinical characteristics may affect the estimation of the arterial path length covered by the pulse propagation using the superficial distance measurement between the neck and the femoral artery. Some of these characteristics are described below.

Age – tortuousness and diameter

As mentioned above, arteries become longer, larger and more tortuous with age, thus the path lengths determined from superficial linear measurements are generally underestimated. The real PWV in the elderly may actually be higher than that calculated by surface-distance measurement [47].

Weight

Overweight subjects, principally men with abdominal obesity, present an increase in abdominal surface. Considering that direct superficial measurement of the distance between the neck and the femoral artery includes the abdominal surface, an overestimation of the superficial measured distance will overcome. Therefore, the real arterial pathway and hence the PWV of obese patients may actually be slightly higher than that calculated using superficial distance measurement.

Breast – bust measurements

As the direct superficial measurement of the distance between the neck and the femoral artery passes over the chest, women with large bust measurements present an overestimation of the real arterial pathway and hence of the PWV. In order to avoid such overestimation, it is recommended that one measures the superficial distance as directly as possible, over the sternum.

Spine – thorax – rib cage

Any marked deformity or morphological abnormality which may affect the spinal column, thorax or rib cage may cause considerable error in the evaluation of the arterial path length from the superficial measurements [47, 59].

In order to determine the effect of these factors, a circulation scheme was arranged by Sands et al. (1924), who analysed these mechanisms in vitro. In the first experiment designed to study the effect of changes in the diameter of the tubes, the walls being constant, they found that the wave velocity is faster in smaller tubes *(table II)*.

TABLE II. Changes in PWV according to the diameter. (Adapted from Sands et al. [47].)

Tube	Diameter (mm)	PWV (m/s)
1	3	16.26
2	4	13.78
3	5	12.54

On the other hand, in tubes where the diameter was constant and the thickness of the wall varied, the velocity was faster with the thicker wall, which is in exact agreement with the formula developed by Moens [11]. To test the effect of twistedness, the tube was threaded through the posts of a test tube rack in such manner as to avoid stretching. The results showed that twisting the tube retards the actual velocity of the wave *(table III)*.

TABLE III. Effects of twistedness on PWV in vitro. (Adapted from Sands et al. [47].)

	Straight tube	Few large turns	Many smaller turns with lumen irregularity
Pulse	13.13	11.91	-
wave	12.24	11.85	9.28
velocity (m/s)	13.90	12.50	11.10

Suggested methods for distance measurements and corrections

■ Subclavian-radial distance

Accurate measurement from the origin of the right subclavian artery to the radial artery at the styloid process can be made by extending the right arm at a 90° angle to the long axis of the body. The length of the subclavian brachio-radial branch can be determined accurately by measuring the direct distance from the sternoclavicular joint to the styloid process of the radius.

■ Subclavian-carotid distance

If the head is not thrown back too far, the carotid vessel can be mapped out with precision from the subclavian artery over the sternoclavicular joint directly to the carotid recording point.

■ Brachial-radial distance

Accurate measurement of the distance from the brachial to the radial artery may be estimated by superficial measurements without specific correction.

■ Femoral-tibial distance

Accurate estimation of the distance from the femoral to the tibial artery may be obtained by direct superficial measurement.

■ Aorta

Some authors suggested that the aortic path length can be estimated from the superficial distance measured between the sternal notch to the level of the umbilicus. Others have suggested measuring the distance between the inferior border of the first left rib just lateral to the midsternal line to the midpoint of a line passing over the iliac crests, and to make a correction for the aortic arch [60].

Aortic arch correction

To make this correction for the arch, 4 cm was added to the measurements in persons over 15 years of age, and 2 cm was added to those of subjects under 15 years. These correction values were obtained from the study of 83 postmortem examinations of persons ranging from three to 99 years of age. The external measurement of the length of the aorta was first made, as described above. After opening the thorax and abdomen, the aorta was carefully cleaned, and the distance from the origin of the left common carotid artery to the bifurcation of the aorta was measured with a piece of string laid carefully along the intima of the aorta. In 47 cases, both the greater and the lesser curvatures of the aorta were measured, and the mean value obtained. In the remaining cases, only the greater curvature was measured. In these, when the greater curvature was measured and compared to the externally measured aortic distance, the average difference was 5.77 cm. In the 47 cases in which both the greater and the lesser curvatures were measured and the mean computed, the average difference between the internally and externally measured distance was 4.87 cm. The average correction factor in the patients under 15 years of age was calculated to be 1.8 cm. For convenience, a correction factor of 2 cm was used in patients under 15 years. Any error due to the use of this factor will be less than ± 4%. While the correction factor actually determined for use above the age of 15 was 4.87 cm, Hallock et al. [60] have added only 4 cm, as the greater part of the postmortem cases in which the correction factor was determined fell in the older age group, and a considerable number of these patients had died of cardiovascular and renal diseases. Any error caused by using this factor of 4 cm will be less than ± 4% in 90% of all cases. In 10% of the cases, error is greater than 4% and may occasionally be as high as 10% [60].

■ Carotid-femoral distance

When pulse waves are recorded from the carotid and femoral arteries, several methods have been described to estimate the arterial path length from superficial distance measurements (see above, arterial path length according to the propagation directions).

Moreover, other authors, in order to determine the carotid-femoral distance, recommended measuring: a) the distance from the lower border of the first left rib to a landmark on the neck (carotid artery); b) the distance from the lower border of the left rib to the midline of the abdomen at the level of the iliac crests; and c) the distance from this latter point to the femoral point. The distance traversed by the pulse wave was calculated as the sum of the two distances (first left rib to midline of the iliac crests plus the midline iliac crests to femoral artery) minus the distance from the first left rib to the carotid site. The same authors suggested adding a correction for the aortic arch (compare with above) [60].

■ Carotid-radial distance

The estimation of the length of this segment of the arterial tree has been computed as the difference between two separate measurements. The first measurement is the distance from the proximal tip of the right clavicle (the usual point of bifurcation of the innominate artery) to the point where the transducer is applied over the right carotid artery; this distance is measured along the right side of the neck, which is slightly extended. The second measurement is the distance from the proximal tip of the right clavicle to the place where the transducer is applied at the styloid process of the radius; this distance is measured along the course of the brachial and radial arteries with the arm extended and the shoulder abducted 90°. Measurements calculated in this fashion were correlated by Bazett and Dreyer to those in the intact cadaver; the error between these two measurements was of the order of 1 cm or less [14].

■ Possible corrections based on anatomic dimensions of the body

Considering the difficulties of estimating the exact arterial length from the superficial distance measurement, several authors have suggested methods for calculating the length of the arteries by measurements between different anatomical landmarks, but these methods are hardly exact. In this regard, and in order to limit the inter-individual anatomical differences of arterial path lengths, thus allowing the comparison of PWV values, Della Corte et al. [59] suggested the introduction of an individual anatomic parameter R, taking into account the different lengths of the aorta and the peripheral arteries. The authors divided the total length into two parts: L_1 = the length between the aortic valves and the bifurcation of the aorta; L_2 = the length from the last point to the peripheral recording points. In order to obtain an estimate of L_1 and L_2, they measured these lengths on thoracic and abdominal aortography of subjects aged between 15 and 70 years without morphological alterations of the aorta. Assuming that PWV values related to L_1 and L_2 are respectively V_1 and V_2, since $V_1 < V_2$, the mean value of the velocity in $L_1 + L_2$ becomes a function of the anatomical ratio R between these two distances: $R = L_2/L_1 + L_2$. In each subject L_1 was assumed to be proportional to the distance (a) between the 7th cervical vertebra and the coccyx, and L_2 to be a linear function of (a) and the distance between the anterior iliac spine and the peripheral site (the calf, in their experience). The length L_1 was found to be a function of age (e) as follows: $L_1 = a (0.002e + 0.72)$; and $L_2 = 0.173 a + b$. As the authors mentioned, this model is a rough approximation [59].

What distance is covered by the carotid-femoral time delay?

Considering that the pulse waves are traveling in the opposite direction throughout the cervical and the aortic-femoral arteries at similar velocities, the covered distance corresponding to the carotid-femoral pulse wave time delay can be calculated from the formula: Velocity (V) = Distance (D) / time-delay (Δt)

$$D = V\Delta t$$

$$D = V (t_F \text{-} t_C)$$

$$D = Vt_F - Vt_C$$

$$D = V(t_F - t_A) - V(t_C - t_A)$$

$$D = D_F - D_C$$

where F corresponds to the aortic-femoral and C to the aortic-cervical pathway *(figure 10)*.

Thus the distance covered by the carotid-femoral pulse wave time delay may be measured by subtracting the distance of the sternal notch (aorta) to the carotid artery from the distance of the sternal notch to the femoral artery *(figure 11)*.

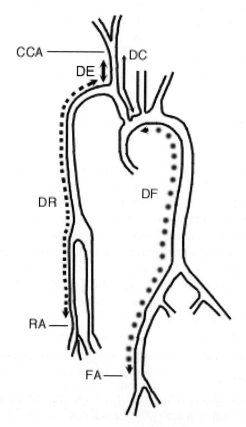

CCA = common carotid artery	DR = distance from the innominate bifurcation artery
FA = femoral artery	to the radial artery
RA = radial artery	DE = distance from the innominate bifurcation artery
DF = distance from the point of emergence	to the carotid artery
of the cervical artery to the femoral artery	DC = distance from the aortic arch to the carotid artery

FIGURE 11. Distance covered by the pulse wave.

What distance is covered by the carotid-radial time delay?

By applying the same consideration of the carotid-femoral pathway, the distance covered by the carotid-radial pulse waves delay is calculated as:

$$D = V\Delta t$$

$$D = V\,(t_R - t_E)$$

$$D = Vt_R - Vt_E$$

$$D = V(t_R - t_E) - V(t_C - t_E)$$

$$D = D_R - D_C$$

where R corresponds to the innominate-radial and E to the innominate-carotid pathway (*figure 11*).

Thus the distance covered by the carotid-radial pulse wave time delay may be measured by subtracting the distance from the proximal tip of the right clavicle (the usual point of bifurcation of the innominate artery) to the carotid artery, from the distance measured between the proximal tip of the right clavicle to the radial artery, measured with the arm extended and the shoulder abducted 90° (*figure 11*).

In summary, despite the use of correction factors, the accuracy of the superficial distance measurement remains limited. Thus, for several reasons (c.f. here above) our recommendation is to perform simple direct measurement of the distance between the two probes.

Patient position and difficulties in pulse wave recordings

■ Patient position

All recordings are usually made from the right side of the body with the patient lying at ease in the supine position. A five to ten minute period of rest has to be given to obtain a steady hemodynamic state. In order to limit measurement variability and allow a reliable comparison between various measurements performed at different times or between different subjects, all patients have to assume as nearly as possible the same position, so that the anatomic landmarks can be easily recognized and accurate measurements taken. The landmarks of the distal part of the common carotid artery can be found by following the superior border of the lamina of the thyroid cartilage out to its very end. At this point, the carotid can most easily be palpated. Because of the anatomic relationships in the neck, it is important that the head be only slightly extended. Excessive extension may introduce an error in measurement [50, 60].

• The radial artery is usually identified by palpation and recorded at the level of the right wrist; the arm is slightly extended and the hand externally rotated.

• The iliac or the femoral arteries are identified by palpating above or below the inguinal ligament; the leg is usually in a slight external rotation position.

• The tibial artery is identified by palpating behind the tibia at the ankle level; the foot is usually in an external rotation position.

• The dorsalis pedis artery may be identified by palpation. Recording of this artery is usually performed using methods based on a nonmechanical transducer, such as ultrasound, photoplethysmography or oscillometric signals.

• The brachial artery is usually identified by palpation and recorded at its maximal prominent part, a few centimetres above the elbow.

• The aortic flow: using a continuous-wave Doppler ultrasound transducer placed in the left supraclavicular fossa pointing medially, some authors recorded the aortic flow close to the origin of the left subclavian artery; others recorded the ascending aortic flow with the transducer placed in the right supraclavicular fossa pointing medially at the front and heart direction.

■ Other difficulties in pulse wave recording

In addition to the above-mentioned difficulties of recording the pulse signals, measuring the distance traveled, and considering the anatomic landmarks, some other factors related to the pulse recording method may be considered.

Influence of applied forces on pulse wave velocity

Influence of applied forces on PWV and transmission in the brachio-radial arterial segment has been investigated recently by Driscoll et al. [61]. The authors hypothesized that PWV, transmission ratios and distal pulse amplitudes may be altered by the recording technique. Brachial and radial arterial pressure pulses were recorded simultaneously using a piezoelectric pulse transducer using ten brachial artery recording forces (0.35 to 3.58 N) applied in a random order and a constant radial force (2.35 N). Pulses were Fourier analysed. Their results showed that in some subjects, the measured variables remained constant until brachial artery recording forces exceeded 2.42 N. The brachial and radial artery recording forces, normally used during clinical measurements, were evaluated in different investigators between 1.23 and 2.10 N. Therefore, at forces normally used by clinical investigators, the PWV, harmonic transmission ratios and pulse amplitudes and contours obtained at the brachial and radial artery are not significantly influenced by forces applied at the brachial artery. However, these variables may be decreased in subjects with more superficial arteries when higher recording forces are used.

In practice, for pressure pulse wave recording, investigators must avoid applying high force, mainly in subjects with superficial arteries.

Extraneous tissue interference

Among the difficulties of pulse wave recording, Klip et al. [56] highlighted the role of extraneous tissue and its interference in PWV measurements. In fact, between the blood, the vessel wall and the sensing transducer, there are tissues, namely the subcutaneous and cutaneous tissues. These tissues function as a tambour with all its inherent bad qualities (amplitude distortion, phase shift and nonlinearity). Hence, the pressure wave may be registered in a distorted form, but this problem makes little difference if the deformation is constant at all registration sites, which is not always the case. In order to limit this difficulty, it is recommended to register the pressure pulse wave at the most prominent and superficial sites, such as the radial and carotid arteries, where the extraneous tissue is limited.

Moreover, even if we assume that the vessel wall and extraneous tissues are constant, deformation would still result from the fact that different harmonics of the pulse wave are propagated with a different velocity; this may give a phase shift and a deformed peripheral curve. Some difficulties inherent within the recording instrument can be reduced by using modern instruments with resonant frequencies greater than 30 cycles/s. At the present time, this latter point is no longer relevant, since all the recording instruments used for manual calculation fulfill these technical requirements and because most of the modern devices now use a computerized acquisition and calculation of algorithms. Elsewhere, Dinnar et al. [62] found that the pressure of the 'viscous' part of the surrounding tissue increases the pulse velocity of the wave over the values found by models, which considered only thick-walled elastic tubes with no surrounding tissue.

Determination of the characteristic point of the wave

The foot or other points?

Conceptually, PWV is determined simply by dividing the distance between two pressure transducers by the time it takes for the wave front to travel between those two points. In practice, determining the wave front is difficult because of changes in pulse contour and amplitude as it propagates. In fact, the pulse wave form changes from the heart to the periphery may be related to several factors: 1) attenuation of the wave as a result of the viscoelastic properties of the arterial wall and viscosity; 2) dispersion of the wave as a result of different traveling velocities of its different frequency components; 3) the wave reflections from peripheral sites, which modify and amplify the pulse wave form; 4) the occurrence of 'natural vibrations' in the arterial tree; and 5) the amplification of the pulse in peripheral arteries as a result of their greater stiffness [34, 63-65].

These modifications of the pulse wave form and contour may affect the diastolic or the systolic parts of the wave but are not usually observed at the beginning of the systole. For this reason, most of the studies using the manual analysis of strip-chart recordings measure the time interval between the wave feet. In fact, the pressure wave foot (i.e., the nadir) is believed to be relatively free of reflections and is the most common point used in locating the wave front.

Since PWV is calculated on the basis of the time interval between the foot of the waves, accurate estimation of this point, which has been referred to as the 'characteristic point', becomes extremely important in PWV measurement. In high-fidelity intra-arterial recordings of pressure, this point can be easily identified as the beginning of the systole initial upstroke or as the minimum diastolic pressure point. When noninvasive methods are used, and manual analysis is performed, this point may not be readily obtained and the foot is determined using an 'intersection' method. Two relatively similar 'intersection' methods have been previously described to estimate the foot point. The first is obtained by the intersection of two tangents, one drawn along the upstroke in early systole and the other through the latter part of the preceding wave diastole; the second method is obtained by the intersection of a line tangent to the wave form pressure initial systolic upstroke and a horizontal line through the minimum point *(figure 12)*; of the two methods, the former has been more widely employed.

Therefore, the foot and the early wave front is a region that maintains its identity in the propagated wave. Extending this idea, Kapal et al. (1951) [45] measured the velocities of four 'corresponding points' on the rising limb and found that they were not appreciably different from each other, thus confirming that the wave front retains its iden-

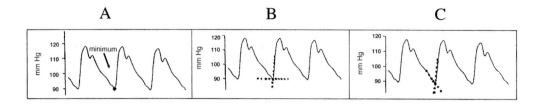

FIGURE 12. Manual determination of the foot or the 'characteristic point' of the pulse wave, using three methods. A = the point of the minimum diastolic pressure. B = intersection of a line tangent to the initial systolic upstroke and a horizontal line through the minimum point. C = intersection of two tangents drawn along the early systolic upstroke and through the latter part of the preceding diastole.

tity reasonably well. This concept was verified in 1968 by McDonald [28], who measured the 'wave front velocity' and showed that the measurement precision depends on the rate of sweep and that the wave front proportion that can be precisely superimposed is about 75% of the wave amplitude in the thoracic aorta and between 30 to 50% in the femoral or more distal arteries. Another identity point of the wave has been checked; the incisura, where it exists, seems to travel at the same velocity as the wave front.

The pulse velocity in the frequency domain

The pressure and flow waves in large arteries are oscillatory. These periodic phenomena can be divided into two components: a steady component, represented by the mean arterial pressure or flow values, and a pulsatile component, which represents the fluctuations or oscillations of blood pressure or flow values around this mean *(figure 13)*. Therefore, for arterial pressure e.g., in addition to the systolic and diastolic values which represent the maximum and minimum points of the pressure curve, other values may be considered: 1) the mean arterial pressure, which is a virtual steady pressure and represents, in a circulation linear model, the applied constant pressure necessary to obtain the same steady flow from a constant pump representing the heart; and 2) the pulse pressure (systolic–diastolic), which represents the blood pressure oscillations amplitude around this mean.

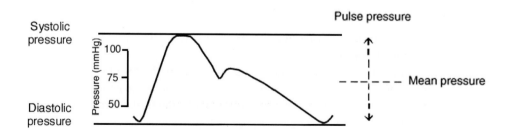

FIGURE 13. Arterial blood pressure wave, considered in terms of its maximum (systolic) and minimum (diastolic) values, and according to the steady component (mean blood pressure) and the amplitude of the oscillations (pulse pressure) around this mean.

This alternative approach to arterial pulse is to consider it as a mean value with oscillations around this mean. Like all oscillatory waves, it can be derived from a series of sine waves and expressed in terms of component = harmonics. This sort of approach is widely employed in the physical sciences, and the technique of deriving series of sine waves from a given pressure or flow wave is the Fourier analysis *(figure 14)*. The harmonic zero reflects the mean value which represents a sine wave with an infinite period, the first harmonic reflects the heart rate, and higher harmonics have a higher frequency. The lower-frequency harmonics of the pulse are always of greater amplitude than the higher harmonics. When all the sine waves are known, their addition leads to the resynthesized original signal from these harmonics. In the cardiovascular system, about 20 harmonics are sufficient for an adequate reconstruction of the blood pressure curve.

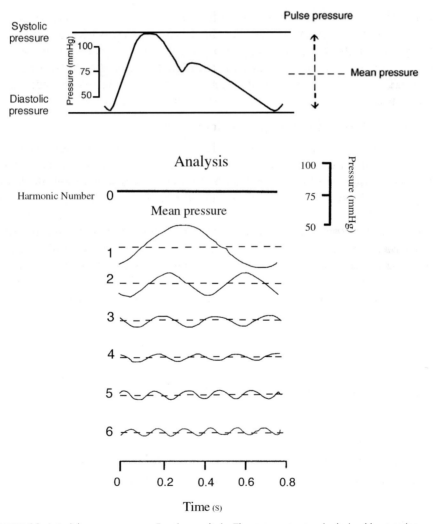

FIGURE 14. Arterial pressure wave, Fourier analysis. The pressure wave is derived by a series of sine waves (harmonics). The harmonic zero represents the mean pressure with an infinite period. The lower-frequency harmonics are of greater amplitude than the higher-frequency harmonics.

Usually, about 98% of the pulse energy is contained in the first five harmonics, and the pulse can be characterized accurately from the first five to ten harmonics [34].

■ Relationship between the phase and the wave front velocity

The harmonic components' velocities showed that phase velocity presents great variations in frequency [34]. This phase velocity is high for components of the pulse below 2 Hz and its fluctuations become very small above 8–10 Hz. This attenuation is mainly related to the reflected waves' attenuation at the higher frequencies *(figure 15)* [28].

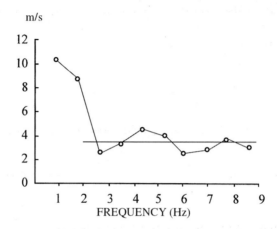

FIGURE 15. Distribution of phase velocities of pulse wave. (Adapted from McDonald, [28].) Velocity is high in low frequencies but the variation above 2 Hz is small. The mean value of the velocities of harmonics above 2 Hz is shown by the solid line; this value coincides with the wave front velocity.

The relatively steady value of phase velocity observed in the higher-frequency components was found by Taylor et al. (1957) to be in good agreement with wave velocities measured from the wave foot [22]. Later on, McDonald (1968) found that the mean value of the phase velocity above 2–2.5 Hz was very close to the wave front velocity [28]. These authors argued that the similarity between the phase velocities, steady value and the foot of the wave velocity is due to the fact that the inflection point is largely determined by the higher-frequency components. Therefore, since the dynamic elastic modulus remains unchanged at frequencies above 2 Hz, the foot value, or the wave front velocity, represents a good measure of the characteristic velocity for all the pulse wave components. Elsewhere, Portaluppi et al. [66] showed that the transmission velocity along the arterial wall is higher for the higher harmonics of the pulse wave (incisura) than for the lower harmonics (upstroke).

More recently, Smulyan et al. [67] recorded the brachial and radial artery pressure curves at different transmural pressures on analogue tape; five pulses were then digitized and subjected to Fourier analysis. The average wave velocity of each of the ten harmonics was calculated and plotted against the harmonic for every transmural pressure. The characteristic wave velocity defined as the average wave velocity of every harmonic was compared with the data obtained for the same beats using the 'hand' method of measurement. Their results showed comparable values and a good agreement between the two methods as expressed by a regression coefficient value of $r = 0.97$ *(figure 16)*.

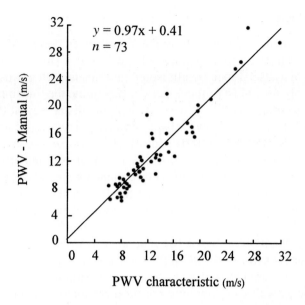

FIGURE 16. Plot of characteristic PWV (PWV) obtained by Fourier analysis vs. PWV obtained by the manual method. (Adapted from Smulyan et al. [67].) Linear regression by the method of least squares.

Taken together, these considerations showed that the wave front velocity, as determined by the upstroke inflection point, represents a good measure of the characteristic velocity for the pulse wave, with a good agreement between the manual and the frequency-analysis methods.

Determination of the time delay between the proximal and the distal front waves

The time delay determination between the 'characteristic' points of the proximal and distal waves can be performed according to several techniques, which may be schematically divided into two major methods: 1) the manual measurements and 2) the automatic determination.

The manual method

After the two pulse wave recordings at high speed, the 'characteristic' point or the wave foot determination can be performed manually, according to different methods (see above). After this determination, two vertical lines are drawn from each of the 'characteristic' points. The interval between these two lines can be directly measured on the recording; this distance interval is then converted to time delay after correction by the paper speed recording: Time Interval = Distance Interval / paper speed. This interval is usually measured for at least ten successive heart beats to cover at least one complete respiratory cycle, and their mean value is considered for the PWV calculation *(figure 10)*.

Automatic devices

Several automatic devices for measuring PWV have been described. They use either a pressure/volume transducer to detect the pulse wave, or a Doppler signal to detect the flow wave or, in one case, a specific ultrasonic instrument with a two-dimensional real-time B-mode [8, 50, 68]. Most of these devices determine the time interval between the foot or the 'characteristic' points of the proximal and distal waves; this is because the foot is relatively free of arterial wave reflections so that interference with the calculation of forward wave velocity is minimized. Many techniques have been proposed for determining the 'characteristic' points: the methods usually performed for the manual calculation, the minimum point, or the intersecting tangents (see above), and the methods usually performed by the automatic devices: the first or the second derivative. In the former, the first derivative of the pulse wave, the point of maximum rate of rise in pressure is usually about halfway up the wave front or somewhat earlier; for the latter, the second derivative, the point at which the second derivative of pressure is maximum is usually around the foot. Karr, in 1982 [69], and Chiu et al. [70], in 1990, have analysed the efficacy of four computerized algorithms in determining time delay and thus the PWV in invasive as well as in noninvasive pressure measurements *(figure 17)*. Their results showed that the 'minimum' point method worked well for the invasive measure-

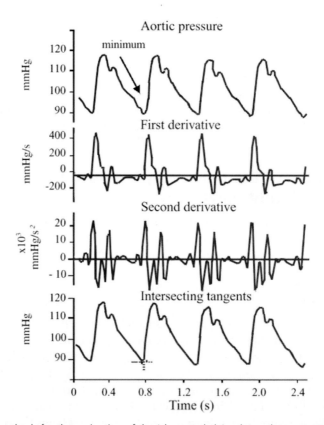

FIGURE 17. Four methods for determination of the 'characteristic' points using computerized algorithms. (Adapted from Chiu et al. [70].) From top to bottom: the 'minimum' point, the maximum first derivative, the maximum second derivative and the intersecting tangents method.

ments, but it was erratic with the noninvasive recordings, probably because of the higher amount of noise; the second derivative and the intersecting tangents methods worked well with both invasive and noninvasive measurements; the first derivative method consistently provided results that were different from the other methods for both the invasive and noninvasive recordings, because of changes in the upstroke contour and structure as the arterial pulse propagates distally. Therefore, if computerized algorithms can be used for automatic PWV determination, it is of a great importance to analyse the accuracy of the method used by its algorithm and to evaluate its determination variability. Since each device has its own and special algorithm, a specific validation must be performed.

In this regard, we analysed the accuracy and reproducibility of the time delay and PWV determination using a recent automatic and computerized device, The Complior® *(figure 12*, chapter I). The results showed good agreement between the manual method (gold standard) and the automatic device with a linear correlation coefficient between the two methods of $r = 0.99$ (automatic = 0.93 manual + 0.56 m/s) *(figure 18)*. The inter-observer and intra-observer repeatability coefficients of PWV measurements using these two methods were found to be > 0.90, thus reflecting highly reproducible measurements *(table IV)* [8, 71].

$n = 56$	Manual method	Complior®	Difference
PWV mean values (m/s) range	11.05 ± 2.58	10.58 ± 2.44	0.20 ± 0.45 (− 0.65,+ 1.26)

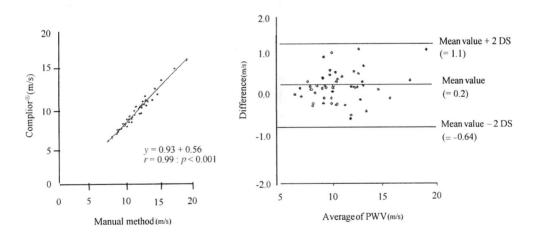

FIGURE 18. Comparison of PWV values performed using the manual method and the Complior® device (validation study adapted from Asmar et al. [50]).

TABLE IV. Inter- and intra-observer reproducibility of PWV measurements
determined using the manual method and the Complior® device. (Adapted from Asmar et al. [8].)

n = 56	Inter-observers		Intra-observer	
	Observer A	Observer B	Time 1	Time 2
PWV. Manual method (m/s)	11.13 ± 2.77	10.98 ± 2.54	11.37 ± 2.77	11.03 ± 2.54
PWV. Complior® device (m/s)	10.96 ± 2.69	10.80 ± 2.39	10.96 ± 2.69	10.77 ± 2.39

AGREEMENT BETWEEN LOCAL AND SEGMENTAL ARTERIAL STIFFNESS

Different noninvasive methods can be used to evaluate arterial stiffness in clinics. Some of these methods assess local arterial wall properties at a single cross-section arterial site, whereas others, e.g., PWV, evaluate arterial stiffness over a specified path length or arterial segment.

Most of the local methods are based on ultrasound, oscillometry or cine-magnetic resonance imaging (MRI) [72]. Usually, these methods assess changes in arterial diameter (or area) between systole and diastole according to the changes in blood pressure [3, 68, 72]. Local measurements are limited by the need to determine blood pressure at the measurement site, something that at present is not feasible in inaccessible arteries, e.g., the aorta. Attempts to overcome this problem by noninvasive means rely on the application of a transfer function to relate either radial or brachial blood pressure to that at the central aorta [34, 63]. On the basis of these measured parameters, changes in local diameter and blood pressure, different and various arterial indexes may be calculated: the cross-sectional compliance, the cross-sectional distensibility, the elastic modulus or more often the beta stiffness index (β index) as described by Kawasaki et al. in 1987 [5]. On the other hand, the 'segmental' methods are based on PWV measurements over a specified arterial path length. Different methods using various signals to detect pulse wave and measure PWV have been reported; based on MRI, ultrasound or more often mechanography, they determine the average stiffness of an arterial segment and do not require the blood pressure at a particular cross section to be known [8, 50, 68].

Few studies have addressed the problem of the comparison between the local and segmental arterial stiffness evaluations. Marque et al. [73] compared in animals the elastic modulus (E) values obtained from the Moens-Korteweg equation using carotid-femoral PWV measurements to those of the incremental elastic modulus Einc calculated from ultrasound assessment of thoracic aortic diameter. Their results showed a significant relationship between the two methods, with systematically lower values of the PWV method. Thus, segmental or static, and local or dynamic properties of the aortic wall evolve in a similar fashion with an agreement between the two methods. More recently, Laurent et al. [74] analysed the relationship between carotid-femoral PWV and carotid dynamic cross-sectional stiffness in hypertensive patients. Their results showed a good agreement between the values of both methods with a coefficient of variation of 6.1% ($r = 0.53$; $p < 0.0001$) and concluded that the classical determinants of arterial stiffness can be shown either with PWV or with dynamic cross-sectional carotid stiffness (figure 19).

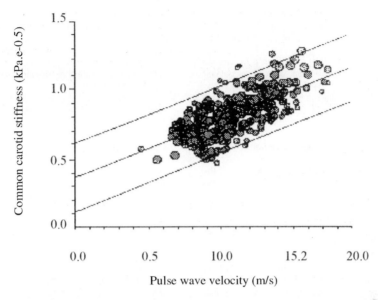

FIGURE 19. Agreement between carotid-femoral PWV and common carotid cross-sectional stiffness. (Adapted from Laurent et al. [71].)

Taken together, these observations suggest that segmental and local arterial stiffness measured at the aortic and carotid levels are in agreement and strongly correlated. Whether similar results may be found in other more peripheral and muscular arterial sites needs to be assessed in specific studies.

REFERENCES

1 Kannel WB. Blood pressure as a cardiovascular risk factor. Prevention and treatment. JAMA 1996 ; 275 : 1571-6.

2 1999 World Health Organization-International society of hypertension guidelines for the management of hypertension. Guidelines sub-committee. J Hypertens 1999 ; 17 : 151-83.

3 Hoeks APG, Brands PJ, Smeets GAM, Reneman RS. Assessment of the distensibility of superficial arteries. Ultrasound Med Biol 1990 ; 16 : 121-8.

4 Tardy Y, Meister JJ, Perret F, Waeber B, Brunner HR. Assessment of the elastic behaviour of peripheral arteries from a non-invasive measurement of their diameter-pressure curves. Clin Phys Meas 1991 ; 12 : 39-54.

5 Kawasaki T, Sasayama S, Yagi SI, Asakawa T, Hirai T. Non-invasive assessment of the age related changes in stiffness of the human arteries. Cardiovasc Res 1987 ; 21 : 678-87.

6 Asmar R, Brunel PC, Pannier BM, Lacolley PJ, Safar ME. Arterial distensibility and ambulatory blood pressure monitoring in essential hypertension. Am J Cardiol 1988 ; 61 : 1066-70.

7 Asmar R, Benetos A, London GM, Hugue C, Weiss Y, Topouchian J, et al. Aortic distensibility in normotensive, untreated and treated hypertensive patients. Blood Pressure 1995 ; 4 : 48-54.

8 Lehman ED, Parker JR, Hopkins KD, Taylor MG, Gosling RG. Validation and reproductibility of pressure-corrected aortic distensibility measurements using pulse-wave velocity Doppler ultrasound. J Biomed Engl 1993 ; 15 : 221-8.

9 Lehmann ED. Pulse wave velocity as a marker of vascular disease. Lancet 1996 ; 348 : 744.

10 Asmar RG, Toupouchian JA, Benetos A, Sayegh FA, Mourad JJ, Safar ME. Non-invasive evaluation of arterial abnormalities in hypertensive patients. J Hypertens 1997 ; 15 Suppl 2 : S99-S107.

11 Moens AI. Die Pulsecurve: Leiden; 1878.

12 Bramwell JC, Hill AV. Velocity of transmission of the pulse wave. Lancet 1922 ; 1 : 891-2.

13 Laubry C, Mougeot A, Giroux R. La vitesse de propagation de l'onde pulsatile artérielle. Arch Mal Cœur 1921 ; 14 : 49-97.

14 Bazett HC, Dreyer NB. Measurements of pulse wave velocity. Am J Physiol 1922 ; 1 : 94-109.

15 Hamilton WF, Remington JW, Dow P. The determination of the propagation velocity of the arterial pulse wave. Am J Physiol 1945 ; 144 : 521.

16 Hamilton WF, Dow P. An experimental study of the standing waves in the pulse propagated through the aorta. Am J Physiol 1939 ; 125 : 48.

17 Korteweg DJ. Ann Phys Chem 1878 ; 241 : 525.

18 Womersley JR. Oscillatory flow in arteries: the reflection of the pulse wave at junctions and rigid inserts in the arterial system. Phys Med Biol 1958 ; 2 : 313-23.

19 Cox RH. Wave propagation through a newtonian fluid contained within a thick-walled, viscoelastic tube. Biophys J 1968 ; 8 : 691-709.

20 Witzig K. Uber erzwungene Wellenbewegungen zaher, inkompressibler Flussigkeiten in elastichen Rohren [Inaugural Dissertation]. Bern, Switzerland: University of Bern; 1952.

21 Morgan GW, Ferrante WR. J Acoust Soc Am 1955 ; 27 : 715.

22 Taylor MG. An experimental determination of the propagation of fluid oscillations in a tube with a visco-elastic wall; together with an analysis of the characteristics required in an electrical analogue. Phys Med Biol 1959 ; 4 : 63-82.

23 Bergel DH. Arterial viscoelasticity. In: Attinger EO, ed. Pulsatile Flow. New York: McGraw-Hill; 1964.

24 Nichols WW, O'Rourke MF, Avolio AP, Yaginuma T, Murgo JP, Pepine CJ, et al. Age-related changes in left ventricular arterial coupling. In: FCP Yin, ed. Ventricular/Vascular Coupling. New York: Springer Verlag; 1987. p. 79-114.

25 Taylor MG. The input impedance of an assembly of randomly branching elastic tubes. Biophys J 1966 ; 6 : 29-51.

26 Bargainer JD. Pulse wave velocity in the main pulmonary artery of the dog. Circ Res 1967 ; 20 : 630-7.

27 Murgo JP, Westerhof N, Giolma JP, Altobelli SA. Aortic input impedance in normal man: relationship to pressure waveforms. Circulation 1980 ; 62 : 10-6.

28 McDonald DA. Regional pulse-wave velocity in the arterial tree. J Appl Physiol 1968 ; 24 : 73-8.

29 Latham RD, Rubal BJ, Westerhof N, Sipkema P, Walsh RA. Nonhuman primate model for regional wave travel and reflections along aortas. Am J Physiol 1987 ; 253 : H299-306.

30 Hess WR. Die Verteilung von Querschnitt, Widerstand, Druckgefalle und Stromungsgeschwindigkeit im Blutfreislauf. Handb d normale u path. Physiol (Bthe) ; Bd. VII, Teil 2. Berlin: Springer Verlag; 1927. p 904-33.

31 Patel DJ, Defreitas FM, Fry DL. Hydraulic input impedance to aorta and pulmonary artery in dogs. J Appl Physiol 1963 ; 18 : 134-40.

32 Learoyd BM, Taylor MG. Alterations with age in the visco-elastic properties of human arterial walls. Circ Res 1966 ; 18 : 278-92.

33 Whitemore RL. Rheology of the Circulation. Oxford: Pergamon; 1968.

34 McDonald DA. Blood flow in arteries: theoretical, experimental and clinical principles. 3rd ed. London: Arnold; 1990.

35 Schmidt-Schonbein H. Microrheology of erythrocytes, blood viscosity, and the distributions of blood flow in the microcirculation. In: International review of physiology. Cardiovascular physiology. Vol 9. Baltimore: University Park Press; 1976. p. 1-62.

36 Hardung V. Propagation of pulse wave in visco-elastic tubing. In: Hamilton WF, Dow P, eds. American Physiological Society Handbook of Physiology, Section 2. Circulation 1961. Vol 1. Washington ; 1962. p 107.

37 Gustafsson L, Appelgren L, Myrvold HE. Effects of increased plasma viscosity and red blood cell aggregation on blood viscosity in vivo. Am J Physiol 1981 ; 241 : H513-8.

38 Stehbens WE. Hemodynamics and the Blood Vessel Wall. Springfield: Charles G. Thomas; 1979.

39 Pannier BM, Safar ME, Laurent S, London GM. Indirect, noninvasive evaluation of pressure wave transmission in essential hypertension. Angiology 1989 ; 40 : 29-35.

40 Avolio AP, Chen SG, Wang RP, Zhang CL, Li MF, O'Rourke MF. Effects of aging on changing arterial compliance and left ventricular load in a northern Chinese urban community. Circulation 1983 ; 68 : 50-8.

41 Luchsinger PC, Snell RE, Patel DJ, Fry DL. Instantaneous pressure distribution along the human aorta. Circ Res 1964 ; 15 : 503-10.

42 Merrillon JP, Fontenier G, Chastre J, Lerallut JF, Jaffrin MY, Gourgon RL. Étude du spectre d'impédance chez l'homme normal et hypertendu. Arch Mal Cœur 1980 ; 73 : 83-90.

43 Latham RD, Westerhof N, Sipkema P, Rubal BJ, Reuderink P, Murgo JP. Regional wave travel and reflections along the human aorta: a study with six simultaneous micromonometric pressures. Circulation 1985 ; 72 : 1257-69.

44 Wezler K, Boger A. Die Dynamik des arteriellen Systems. Der Arterielle Blutdruck und seine Komponenten. Ergebn Physiol 1939 ; 41 : 292-306.

45 Kapal E, Martini F, Wettere E. Uber die Zuverlassigkeit der bisherigen Bestimmungsart der Pulswellen geschwindigkeit. Z Biol 1951 ; 104 : 75-86.

46 Zangeneh, Nassereslami. Z Kreisl-Forsch 1967 ; 56 : 368.

47 Sands J. Studies in pulse wave velocity in pathological conditions. Am J Physiol 1925 ; 71 : 519-33.

48 Milnor WR, Conti CR, Lewis KB, O'Rourke MF. Pulmonary arterial pulse wave velocity and impedance in man. Circ Res 1969 ; 25 : 637-49.

49 Caro CG, McDonald DA. The relation of pulsatile pressure and flow in the pulmonary vascular bed. J Physiol 1961 ; 157 : 426-53.

50 Asmar R, Benetos A, Topouchian J, Laurent P, Pannier B, Brisac AM, et al. Assessment of arterial distensibility by automatic pulse wave velocity measurement. Validation and clinical application studies. Hypertension 1995 ; 26 : 485-90.

51 Mackay RS, Marg E, Oechsli R. Automatic tonometer with exact theory: various biological applications. Science 1960 ; 131 : 1688-9.

52 Kelly R, Hayward C, Ganis J, Daley J, Avolio A, O'Rourke M. Non-invasive registration of the arterial pressure pulse waveform using high-fidelity applanation tonometry. J Vasc Med Biol 1989 ; 3 : 142-9.

53 Gosling RG. Extraction of physiological information from spectrum-analysed Doppler-shifted continuous-wave ultrasound signals obtained non-invasively from the arterial system. IEE Med Electr Monogr 1976 ;18 : 73-125.

54 Avolio AP, Fa-Quan D, Wei-Qian G L, Yao-Fei L, Zhen-Dong H, Lian-Fen X, et al. Effects of aging on arterial distensibility in populations with high and low prevalence of hypertension : comparison between urban and rural communities in China. Circulation 1985 ; 71 : 202-10.

55 Benthin M, Dahl P, Ruzicka R, Lindström K. Calculation of pulse wave velocity using cross correlation - Effects of reflexes in the arterial tree. Ultrasound Med Biol 1991 ; 17 : 461-9.

56 Klip W. Difficulties in the measurement of pulse-wave velocity. Am Heart J 1958 ; 6 : 806-13.

57 Lehman ED, Gosling RG, Fatemi-Langroudi B, Taylor MG. Non-invasive Doppler ultrasound technique for the in vivo assessment of aortic compliance. J Biomed Engl 1992 ; 14 : 250-6.

58 Beyerholm O. Studies of the velocity of transmission of the pulse wave in normal individuals. Acta Med Scand 1927 ; 67 : 203.

59 Della Corte M, Locchi F, Spinelli E, Scarpelli PT. Effect of the anatomical structure of the arterial tree on the measurement of pulse wave velocity in man. Phys Med Biol 1979 ; 24 : 593-9.

60 Hallock P. Arterial elasticity in man in relation to age as evaluated by the pulse wave velocity method. Arch Int Med 1934 ; 54 : 770-98.

61 Driscoll MD, Arnold JM, Marchiori GE, Sherebrin MH. Influence of applied brachial recording forces on pulse wave velocity and transmission in the brachio-radial arterial segment. Clin Invest Med 1995 ; 18 : 435-48.

62 Dinnar U. The role of the surrounding tissue in the propagation of waves through the arterial system. TIT J Life Sci 1975 ; 5 : 49-56.

63 Kelly R, Hayward C, Avolio A, O'Rourke M. Noninvasive determination of age-related changes in the human arterial pulse. Circulation 1989 ; 80 : 1652-9.

64 O'Rourke MF, Kelly RP. Wave reflection in the systemic circulation and its implications in ventricular function. J Hypertens 1993 ; 11 : 327-37.

65 Safar ME, Frohlich ED. The arterial system in hypertension. A prospective view. Hypertension 1995 ; 26 : 10-4.

66 Portaluppi F, Knighten V, Luisada AA. Transmission delays of different portions of the arterial pulse. A comparison between the indirect aortic and carotid pulse tracings. Acta Cardiol 1983 ; 38 : 49-59.

67 Smulyan H, Csermely TJ, Mookherjee S, Warner RA. Effect of age on arterial distensibility in asymptomatic humans. Arteriosclerosis 1983 ; 3 : 199-205.

68 Benthin M, Dahl P, Ruzicka R, Lindström K. Calculation of pulse–wave velocity using cross correlation-effects of reflexes in the arterial tree. Ultrasound Med Biol 1991 ; 17 : 461-9.

69 Karr SG. Theoretical and experimental determination of arterial pulse propagation speed [dissertation]. Evanston (Ill): Northwestern University; 1982.

70 Chiu YC, Arand PW, Schroff SG, Feldman T, Carroll JD. Determination of pulse wave velocities with computerized algorithms. Am Heart J 1991 ; 121 : 1460-70.

71 Laurent P. Étude de la vitesse de propagation de l'onde de pouls : de la recherche expérimentale à la pratique clinique [thèse]. Université de Bordeaux ; 1994.

72 Bolster BD Jr, Atalar E, Hardy CJ, McVeigh ER. Accuracy of arterial pulse wave velocity measurement using MRI. J Magn Reson Imaging 1998 ; 8 : 878-88.

73 Marque V, VanEssen H, Struyker-Boudier HAJ, Atkinson J, Lartaud-Idjouadiène I. Comparison of aortic elastic modulus determined by echo-tracking and pulse wave velocity. Workshop "Arterial Structure, and Function", Versailles, France. January 1998.

74 Laurent S, Boutouyrie P. Agreement between aortic stiffness determined as carotid-femoral pulse wave velocity (PWV) and carotid stiffness determined as dynamic cross-sectional stiffness, in hypertensive patients. Workshop "Arterial Structure, and Function", Versailles, France. January 1998.

IV

CHAPTER

Factors influencing pulse wave velocity

The velocity with which the pulse wave is transmitted is dependent primarily on the coefficient of elasticity or rigidity of the artery. However, several other factors deserve consideration. Some of these factors are related to cardiovascular physiology, others are consecutive with pathophysiological conditions. The purpose of this chapter is to describe the factors influencing PWV, its modifications in various situations and its relations with different hemodynamic and biochemical factors.

AGE

(See also chapter V, section on Atherosclerosis.)

Age and arteriosclerosis affect the arterial tree differently; their corresponding alterations predominate in the central and elastic arteries and therefore modify in different manners the central and peripheral PWV [1]. In fact, since the beginning of this century, it appears that alterations that occur with age, especially in the aorta, involve corresponding regressive changes in the elastic tissue. Aschoff in 1924 [2] called attention to the fact that when an aorta was loosened from its attachments from the vertebral column, except at its ends, and then cut transversely through its midportion, the cut ends would retract considerably in young people, but not to any appreciable extent in older subjects. He attributed this difference to weakening of the elastic tissue. With advancing age, the size of the aorta gradually increases, and physical tests indicate that extensibility decreases. Later on, Zon (1932), in an attempt to correlate the physical behavior of aortas at various ages with their respective histologic structures, determined the extensibility of rings of aortas from all periods of life [3]. His study showed a progressive disappearance of elastic tissue with a slight replacement by collagenous tissue and a change in form of the elastic fibres with age. Hence, he expressed the belief that the decrease of extensibility with age is due to the degeneration of elastic tissue. Numerous more recent experiments and studies using more or less sophisticated approaches corroborate these results [4, 5]. From all the preceding considerations, it is obvious that the factors which govern the transmission of the pulse wave and its velocity in medium- and small-sized vessels are not altogether similar to those that govern its transmission in aortas and large-sized arteries.

Age and central (trunk or aortic) pulse wave velocity

Numerous population studies showed that values of aortic PWV (or carotid-femoral or trunk PWV) increase with age in both sexes. Hallock et al. [6] described the dispersion of mean values for the aortic PWV as essentially constant for both sexes up to about 40 years, after which it increases rapidly. Differences between the mean aortic PWV values observed for successive age groups (classified by five- or ten-year periods) of both sexes have been described as significant *(figure 1)*.

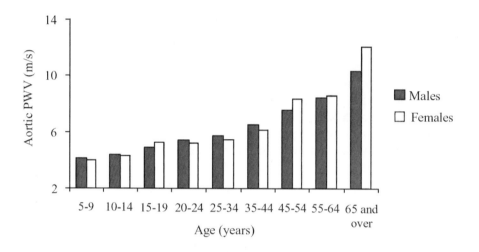

FIGURE 1. Age changes in the aortic PWV of both sexes. (Adapted from Hallock et al. [6].)

The effect of age and sex on in vivo arterial wall compliance has been also analysed by Laogun et al. [7], who showed that in vivo aortic compliance increases sharply with age in the first decade of life, reaching a peak at around ten years, thereafter decreasing with age (more in males than females until the 50-year range); for these authors, it is not only the distensibility of the artery that is important but also the stage of life at which it is observed [7].

More recent studies using noninvasive techniques based on blood flow velocity [7-9] or pressure waves [10-12] to assess PWV showed that advancing age causes an increase in aortic or carotid-femoral PWV. A number of these studies have analysed the effect of age on aortic PWV using multiple regression analysis or other methodological aspects (matched population), which take into consideration the different determinants of PWV affected by age, such as blood pressure, heart rate, etc. Their results were in agreement and highlighted age as a major determinant of aortic PWV. Similar results have been reported in several populations in different countries [9] *(figures 2, 3)*. We analysed the determinants of the carotid-femoral PWV in the untreated hyper-

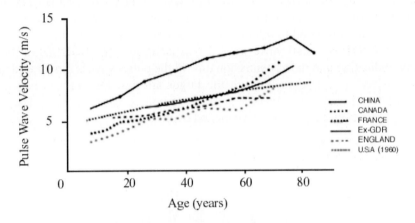

FIGURE 2. Relation between PWV and age in different countries. (Adapted from Avolio [9].)

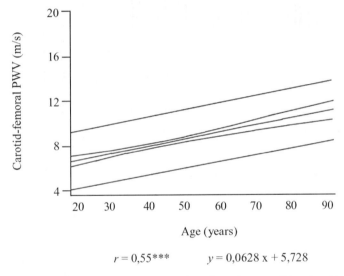

$$r = 0{,}55^{***} \qquad y = 0{,}0628\,x + 5{,}728$$

FIGURE 3. Linear correlation between PWV and age in normal French subjects. Normograph and its confidence intervals. (Adapted from Asmar et al. [11].)

tensive patients of the Complior® study performed in about 2,000 patients from 19 countries (personal data). The results showed age as a major determinant, followed by systolic blood pressure [13].

Age and peripheral pulse wave velocity

Peripheral PWV can be measured in the upper limbs (carotid-radial, brachial-radial) or lower limbs (femoro-tibial). In order to understand cardiovascular physiopathology, it is important to analyse the effect of age on PWV not only in the aorta but also in the peripheral arteries. In this regard, numerous population studies have described these relationships principally at the level of the upper limbs and to a lesser extent in the lower limbs.

Early in this century, Bramwell and Hill [22], Hallock et al. [6], and Beyerholm [14] showed a progressive increase in the velocity of the arm pulse waves with age, from a value of 5.1 in mid-childhood to 6.3 m/s at 22 years of age and to 9.6 m/s at 65 years of age. The velocity of the radial pulse wave is consistently higher than that of the aortic pulse wave, indicating that the transmission time of the pulse wave is more rapid through the medium-sized vessels than through the larger arteries. Differences between age groups (classified by five- or ten-year periods) of both sexes have been described as significant except from the age of 65 years and over *(figures 4, 5)*.

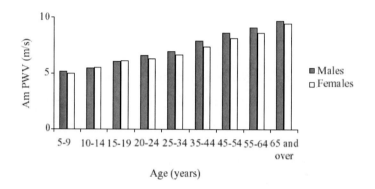

FIGURE 4. Age changes in the arm (carotid-radial) PWV of both sexes.
(Adapted from Hallock et al. [6].)

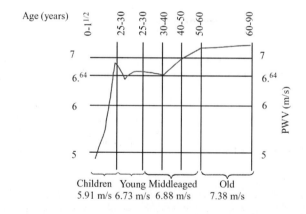

FIGURE 5. Changes of carotid-radial PWV with age. (Adapted from Beyerholm [14].)

Different effects of age on central and peripheral arteries

In order to assess the effects of age on different arteries and to verify whether age affects in a different manner the central and peripheral arteries, several studies analysed the effects of age on different arterial sites in the same patients. Moreover, in order to minimize the age-related effects of atherosclerosis and thus to analyse the effects of age per se on arterial stiffness, studies have been conducted in populations with a known low prevalence of atherosclerosis. In this regard, Avolio et al. [8, 9] measured PWV in a Chinese population at three different levels: the aorta, the arm and the leg, and found that central PWV is generally lower than peripheral PWV but increases to a greater degree with age according to the following equations between PWV (y – cm/s) and age (x – years):

- aorta: $y = 9.2\ x + 615$; $r = 0.673$,
- arm: $y = 4.8\ x + 998$; $r = 0.453$,
- leg: $y = 5.6\ x + 791$; $r = 0.630$ (figure 6).

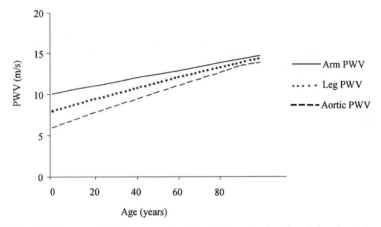

FIGURE 6. Changes of pulse wave velocities in the central and peripheral arteries with age in urban Chinese population. (Adapted from Avolio et al. [8].)

These results corroborate previous data observed in population studies as described by Hallock et al. [6] (figure 7).

More recently, Benetos et al. [1] assessed the effects of age on local cross-sectional distensibility coefficients at the carotid and femoral arteries of the same subjects. Their results showed that whereas age was strongly correlated with arterial distensibility at the site of the carotid artery, no significant correlation was observed at the femoral artery (figure 8).

In summary, these observations taken together showed an increase in arterial stiffness and PWV with age. This increase of PWV with age is more pronounced in central elastic arteries than in peripheral muscular arteries. These changes have been described in different populations and using different methodological aspects to be independent of any increase of blood pressure or other age-related parameters [1-17]. In the aorta, the greatest change appears to be between ages ten and 50, with an approximate increase of 60%, whereas in the peripheral arteries the change is far less, with an almost 20% increase in both the arm and leg. These results indicate that noninvasive PWV measurements tend to an equivalent value in the central and peripheral arteries in subjects aged over 60 years (figures 6, 7). These observations are in agreement with the greater propensity and

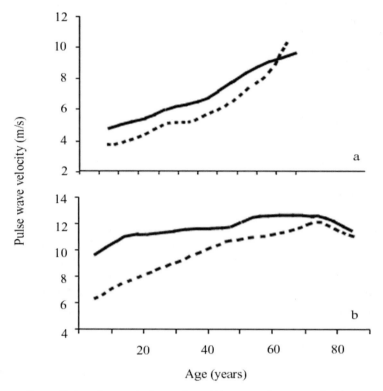

FIGURE 7. Age changes in the aortic and the arm pulse wave velocities
(**a:** adapted from Hallock et al. [6]; **b:** from Avolio et al. [8]); (—) arm PWV, (– – –) aortic PWV.

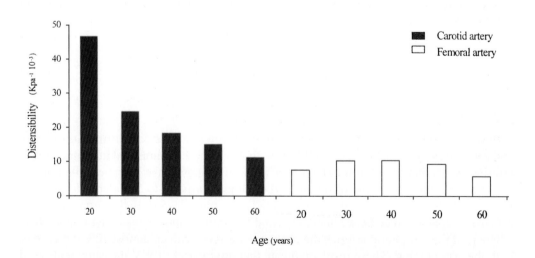

FIGURE 8. Effects of age on carotid and femoral distensibility coefficients in the same subjects.
(Adapted from Benetos et al. [1].)

incidence of atherosclerosis in the central large arteries, such as the aorta and its first collateral arteries.

BLOOD PRESSURE

(See also chapter V, section on Hypertension.)

As long ago as 1878, Moens [18] showed that the elasticity of the blood vessels as measured by PWV varied with the blood pressure. Grunmach [19], shortly after this (1885), confirmed his observations and also showed that the PWV might show considerable variations with blood pressure in man. Dawson [20], however, in 1917, investigated in animals the relationship between blood pressure and PWV and found no consistent relationships between them. This result, in reality, is not surprising since the correlations between these two parameters differ significantly whether we consider central or peripheral arterial pulse wave and whether we analyse systolic, diastolic, mean or pulse pressure. In fact, with vessels having pronounced histologic and pathophysiological differences, as do the various arteries, it is not to be expected that their elasticity will depend only–according to a constant relationship–on their pressure; this, though, is likely to be one variable factor, and consequently such described discrepancies may be expected. Attention to such considerations has been discussed since 1922 by Bramwell et al. [21, 22]. The authors described a method by which the extensibility of the brachio-radial artery could be measured at all internal pressures from zero up to the diastolic pressure in a living man. By the employment of a compression bandage they were able to modify the effective pressure inside a certain region of an artery and to calculate the PWV in the segment of artery submitted to various pressures, making use of the formula: $PWV = d / y - x (1 - d)/l$, in which x equals the transmission time between two points at a distance l from each other, and y the time between the same points when a bandage of length d is applied. They found that the velocity of the pulse wave increased and therefore extensibility decreased as the intra-arterial pressure was increased. By an ingenious method, the same investigators experimentally confirmed these deductions by direct mechanical measurements of the velocity of the pulse wave in isolated arteries which were filled with mercury in order to slow the transmission of the wave. Their results indicated conclusively that the velocity of the pulse wave increased almost as directly as the blood pressure, and that the rate of propagation of the pulse wave was a mechanical phenomenon depending on the elastic properties of the vessels. Thus with increasing diastolic pressure there appeared to be a gradual increase of rigidity *(figure 9)*. Later on, the same investigators repeated their experiences on an isolated carotid artery and converted their above-mentioned formula into another convenient form, where the PWV may be expressed in terms of millimetres of mercury rise of pressure per 1% increase of volume, or rigidity of the artery as follows:

$$PWV = 3.57 \sqrt{\frac{\text{mmHg of pressure}}{\text{required to produce 1\% increase in volume}}}$$

Since in the Bramwell et al. study [22], the whole of the arm under the bandage was subjected to pressure, it is possible that factors other than pressure changes within the

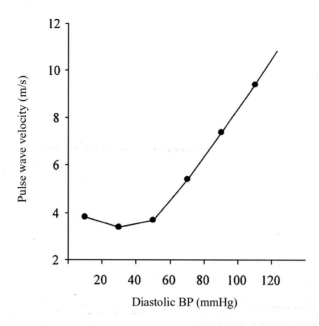

FIGURE 9. Relationship between diastolic BP and PWV.
(Adapted from Bramwell and Hill, figures on excised carotid [22].)

artery might have contributed to the results. In order to eliminate these external factors and to obtain a localised change of blood pressure in one artery, Hickson et al. [23] analysed the effect of the arm position on PWV. In their study, subjects remained in the same position, the right arm being passively raised or lowered. In all cases, a fall in systolic blood pressure of 20-30 mmHg when the arm was raised above the head from the horizontal position with a lengthening of the carotid-radial time interval was observed with an appreciable slowing of the PWV.

At the same time, Bazett et al. [24], considering the relative accuracy of the auscultatory method for the diastolic BP determination (phase IV of Korotkoff sounds), analysed the relationship of blood pressure to the pulse wave velocities. They plotted their results against systolic, diastolic and mean pressures, estimating the latter as "both at midway between the systolic and diastolic pressure and also nearer the diastolic pressure," taking it as equal to the diastolic pressure plus one-third of the pulse pressure. They found with the mean blood pressure that the figures comparing carotid and radial pulses seemed to give the best agreement, and assumed that mean BP was the pressure to be taken into consideration with the PWV. Later on, Sands et al. [25] suggested that the correlations which occur between blood pressure and PWV may differ according to the arterial wall condition and state. They found that the described correlation between PWV and diastolic BP in normal subjects may be lost in patients with arterial abnormalities, and described in various pathophysiological figures better correlations with systolic than diastolic pressure. They suggested that factors such as 'hardening of the arterial wall' and arterial wall 'muscular contraction' modify PWV in normal and abnormal subjects, so that diastolic pressure is not the dominant factor. From their experience, it appeared that in normal subjects, PWV correlates about equally well with systolic or diastolic pressure, whereas in abnormal figures, these correlations are considerably modified.

Moreover, according to Steele et al. [26], among the variables which relate speed of pulse wave to elasticity, blood pressure is important to consider not only because it exerts a great effect upon the speed of the pulse wave but also because its physiological variations are rapid, frequent and large. For these authors, when velocity is used as an index of distensibility, the pressure at which it is measured is then important. Among the systolic, diastolic and mean pressures, they state that it is obvious that diastolic BP is the most important because: 1) it is the pressure at which the pulse wave is transmitted since velocity is customarily calculated by measurements made upon the first upstroke of the pulse wave, the one which begins at the diastolic level of pressure; 2) as shown by Wiggers [27], the pressure waves produced at the systolic level travel at higher speeds than those ordinarily recorded for pulse wave transmission; and 3) as demonstrated by Frank [28], reflected waves do not appear upon the pulse wave soon enough to disturb the initial upstroke beginning at diastolic levels of pressure. It is important to note here that Steele's interpretation of these arguments is confused; in fact, it is not because measurements are made upon the first upstroke, which is not usually affected by the reflected waves, that the velocity of the pulse wave should not be related to other blood pressures than diastolic. Furthermore, the usual reason for correlating the PWV with various pressure levels appears to be that in dealing with large groups of individuals (in contrast to most of the above cited experiences), several authors have been unable to find a correlation with the diastolic level.

Other factors such as arteriolar resistance, cardiac output, blood volume and blood viscosity being constant, the less elastic the arteries, the higher the systolic and pulse pressures will be, the more the work of the heart, and the less uniform capillary blood flows. Considering these factors, Haynes et al. [29] analysed the relationship of PWV to blood pressure in patients with hypertension, arteriosclerosis and related conditions and complications. Their results showed a close correlation between pulse pressure and PWV with a stronger correlation with the aortic (such as the subclavian-femoral) PWV than with the arm or leg pulse wave velocities. According to these authors, in general, as the extensibility decreases (i.e., as the velocity increases, whether due to arterial change or to increased pressure), the pulse pressure increases (figure 10).

All these studies performed at the beginning of the 20th century showed that blood pressure may influence PWV to a greater extent than the anatomical nature of the vessel walls and the dimensions of the arteries. Observations on human beings analysing whether the velocity is related to systolic, diastolic, mean or pulse pressures varied considerably. However, as has been pointed out by Hallock [6], certain (if not the majority) of these studies are not valid, since several aspects of the methodology used can be criticised, and in most of them the age factor has not been eliminated. In fact, PWV increases with advancing age, closely following the rise in blood pressure which occurs as one grows older; one would expect to find a rise in PWV with a rise in blood pressure. In order to consider age, and since varying correlation coefficients have been reported between the various pulse wave velocities (aorta–leg–arm) and blood pressures (systolic, diastolic, mean, pulse), population studies have been performed. Eliakim et al. [30] found higher values in hypertensive subjects only after age 60. Schimmler et al. found

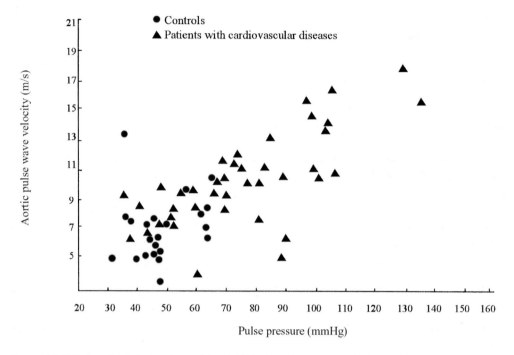

FIGURE 10. Relation of subclavian-femoral (aortic) PWV to pulse pressure. (Adapted from Haynes et al. [29].)

in German populations [15] a definite increase in aortic PWV with mean arterial pressure at all ages *(figure 11)*, whereas a less definite relationship was found by Avolio et al. [8] in Chinese subjects, and Ho et al. in an Australian community, where age was the main determinant. In their study, Ho et al. [31] showed that aortic PWV (brachio-

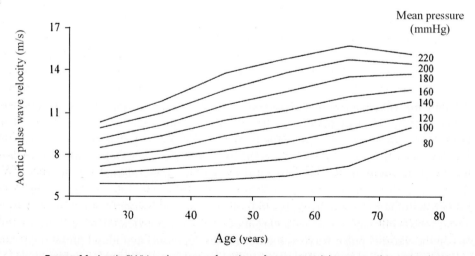

FIGURE 11. Aortic PWV and age as a function of mean arterial pressure determined from external recordings of carotid and femoral pulses. (Adapted from Schimmler et al. [15].)

cephalic and femoral arteries) rose with age and was also related to arterial pressure, but both PWV and blood pressure increase with age; when compared at different ages, there was no statistically significant difference in PWV at different pressures. These different results may be due to the relatively small numbers of subjects in the respective sub-groups of age and blood pressure.

More recent studies performed in untreated large populations of normotensives and hypertensives with a large age range and without any cardiovascular disease analysed the determinants of PWV according to an adequate statistical approach. Their results are in agreement and showed that the major determinants of PWV are age and systolic blood pressure. For the central PWV (carotid-femoral), age was the main determinant, whereas for the peripheral pulse wave velocities (arm–leg), the role of blood pressure dominated. According to this approach, the following regression equations were observed for the carotid-femoral PWV in a French population and its normotensive and hypertensive subgroups [10, 11]:

– population: PWV (m/s) = 0.07 systolic BP (mmHg) + 0.09 age (years) – 4.3

– normotensive subjects: PWV (m/s) = 0.06 systolic BP (mmHg) + 0.09 age (years) – 2.3

– hypertensive subjects: PWV (m/s) = 0.06 systolic BP (mmHg) + 0.09 age (years) – 2.7

The higher correlation coefficient between carotid-femoral PWV and blood pressure in this population study was noted with systolic BP; such observations may be easily expected since the major determinant of systolic blood pressure is known to be the distensibility of the large artery, as evaluated by the carotid-femoral PWV.

Influence of the method of BP measurements

As mentioned above, varying correlation coefficients have been reported between PWV and the different arterial pressures (systolic, diastolic, etc.). This variation may be attributable, at least in part, to the inherent variability in both PWV and blood pressure within and across individual subjects. Since blood pressure is a hemodynamic parameter with high short-term and long-term variabilities, the method of its measurements may greatly influence the observed relations between blood pressure and PWV. Elsewhere, several studies have shown that repeated measurements of blood pressure and ambulatory BP monitoring provide a better time integral of the strain exerted on the heart and vessels. Thus, it is now well established that ambulatory BP monitoring correlates more strongly than clinical BP with indexes of target organ damage in hypertensives. In order to analyse the relationships between carotid-femoral PWV and blood pressure in hypertensive patients, we determined the blood pressure level using three different methods: casual measurement performed by the practitioner, automatic BP monitoring in a clinic (Dinamap device) with one measure every three minutes during 30 minutes, and 24-hour ambulatory BP monitoring [32]. The results concerning the relationship between PWV and BP level differed according to the method used. Significant correlations were observed with the BP monitoring in clinic (Dinamap) and the 24-hour ambulatory monitoring, though not with the casual measurements. For the clinical monitoring, the only significant correlation was observed with systolic BP, whereas for the 24-hour ambulatory monitoring, significant correlations were observed with both systolic and mean BP: the best correlations were noticed with the daytime values *(table I)*. These results showed that the relationship between PWV and BP level is influenced by the method of BP measurement; serial BP monitoring in a clinic or under ambulatory conditions is more sensitive than casual BP measurements for evaluating this relationship; PWV is correlated with systolic BP and to a lesser extent with mean BP measured over the day-time period in hypertensive patients.

TABLE I. Correlation coefficients between carotid-femoral PWV and blood pressure and heart rate values measured with different methods in hypertensive subjects. (Adapted from Asmar et al. [32].)

	Casual BP measurement	Dinamap monitoring (30 minutes)	Ambulatory monitoring		
			24 hours	Daytime	Nighttime
Systolic BP (mmHg)	0.241	0.453*	0.624**	0.685***	0.320
Diastolic BP (mmHg)	0.221	0.369	0.340	0.360	0.155
Mean BP (mmHg)	0.138	0.399	0.474*	0.507*	0.232
Heart rate (beat/min)	0.117	− 0.118	0.358	0.469*	0.031

$*p < 0.05$; $** p < 0.01$; $*** p < 0.001$

In summary, taken together these considerations showed close correlations between the PWV and blood pressure level, which constitute an independent determinant of PWV. These correlations have been reported with the different blood pressures: systolic, diastolic, mean or pulse pressure; the highest correlation coefficients were noted frequently with systolic BP. This relationship between PWV and BP is influenced by the method of BP measurements, the strongest correlation being observed using serial BP measurements under ambulatory conditions. Using an adequate statistical approach, BP has been shown as the major determinant for central PWV, but also to a greater extent for peripheral pulse wave velocities. Based on these observations, determining radial blood pressures from PWV measurements has been recently proposed and constitutes one of the research fields for noninvasive BP determination.

GENDER

(See also first section on Age, and chapter V, section on Postmenopausal women.)

Bazett et al. [24], in 1922, after investigating PWV in a small group of normal subjects, concluded that "it seems probable that the values in young adult females are rather lower than those in males." Because of the small number of subjects, the authors did not draw any positive conclusions. Beyerholm [14], in 1927, analysed PWV in normal individuals and the comparison between males and females showed an average PWV value greater in male than in female individuals in the various age groups, except as regards those of children and old people (> 60 years). For the author, "it must be justifiable to conclude that PWV, at any rate in the young age, is a little greater in males than in females, about 5%." No definite conclusion was given regarding the children's and old persons' groups. Hallock [6], in 1937, reported that the velocity of the aortic pulse wave in males exceeds that in females, except in the age period between 15 and 19 years, whereas the aortic PWV in females exceeds that in males after the age of 45 years *(figure 12)*. Loagun et al. [7] showed that aortic compliance (derived from PWV) increases sharply in the first decade of life, and decreases after another ten years more in males than in females until the 50-year-old range *(figure 13)*. Sonesson et al. [33] analysed arterial stiffness at the level of the distal abdominal aorta in healthy females and males aged from four to 74 years; their results showed an increase of aortic stiffness with age which was linear in females and greater and exponential in males, suggesting that degenerative changes appear later in females than in males. London et al. [34] investigated normotensive and hypertensive subjects with no history of cardiovascular disease; their results showed: 1) in premenopausal women, lower values of PWV were measured at the upper-limb and lower-limb levels than in age-matched men, whereas aortic PWV was not different; and 2) in postmenopausal women, there were similar values for the three measured pulse wave velocities to that of age-matched men *(figure 14)*. More recently, we analysed the determinants of carotid-femoral PWV in 1,810 untreated hypertensive patients from the

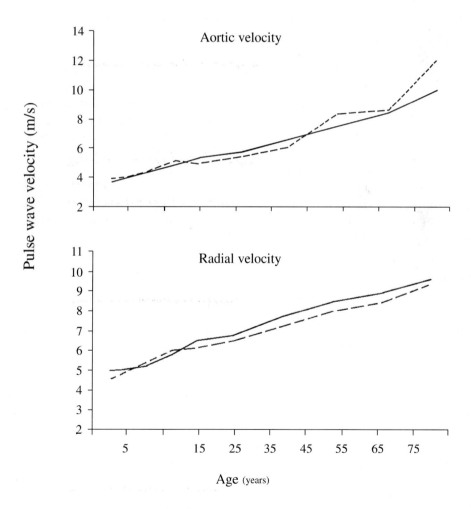

FIGURE 12. Progressive increase of the aortic and the arm pulse wave velocities for males and females with age (adapted from Hallock [6]); (—) male, (–·–) female.

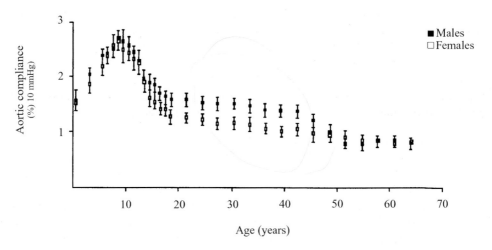

FIGURE 13. Variations of aortic compliance, calculated on the basis of PWV measurements, with age and sex. (Adapted from Laogun et al. [7].)

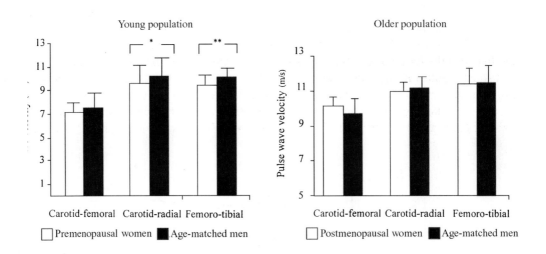

FIGURE 14. PWV in normotensive premenopausal and postmenopausal women by comparison to age-matched men. (Adapted from London et al. [34].)

Complior® study (974 males, 836 females); the results showed higher pulse wave, adjusted for age, in men than in women (personal data) [13].

In summary, numerous studies performed in healthy individuals or under pathological conditions showed, as a rule, higher PWV in men than in women at adult and middle age, whereas similar values have been suggested in children and the elderly.

HEART RATE

Several studies have analysed the effect of heart rate on PWV, principally in terms of linear correlation between the two variables. Before reporting their results, it is important to note here that different techniques have been variously used in these studies to evaluate PWV: by measuring the time intervals between the outset of the QRS (ECG) complex and the outset of a peripheral pulse wave, or of the time intervals between two peripheral pulse waves recorded simultaneously. These are obviously not comparable, since the former includes time consumed for intracardiac events.

Early studies have suggested that heart rate has no effect on PWV [14]. Sands et al. [25] in a series of experiments designed to analyse the effect of change of pulse wave rate on the velocity did not show any significant difference; for example, the wave velocity at a wave rate of 92 per minute was 13.38 m/s, while at 150 per minute it was 13.52 m/s. Eliakim et al. [30] have analysed the effect of a changing pulse rate on the femoral-pedis PWV according to two methods of measuring the time periods: 1) between the feet of the pulse waves of the femoral and the dorsalis pedis arteries; and 2) between the QRS complex and the pulse wave of the dorsalis pedis artery. They studied subjects with persistent A-V block (second and third degrees) who where being treated by external transvenous pacemakers. In some patients, PWV was measured during the slow spontaneous A-V nodal rhythm and again during pacing at a fixed rate of about 75 beats/min. In other patients, measurements of PWV were made during pacing of rates varying between a minimum of 48 to 67 and a maximum of 103 to 156 per minute. Their results showed that in patients with A-V block, the wave velocity measured between the feet of the pulse waves showed no significant change when values during a spontaneous rate were compared with values during pacing at a fixed rate of 60 per minute or at increasing fixed rates. An illustrative example is given in *figure 15*. Elsewhere, contradictory results have been reported from experimental studies. Callaghan et al. [35] reported in isolated canine common carotids assessed at different pulse fre-

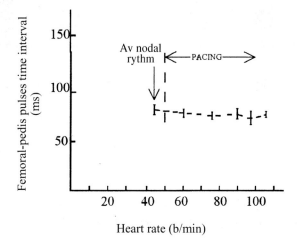

FIGURE 15. Relationship between pulse rate and PWV as measured between the feet of the pulse waves of femoral and dorsalis pedis arteries in a patient with complete heart block, before and after pacing at different rates. No change was noted by pacing. (Adapted from Eliakim et al. [30].)

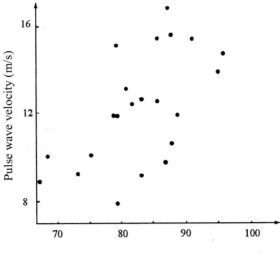

FIGURE 16. Relationship between carotid-femoral PWV
and ambulatory daytime heart rate values. (Adapted from Asmar et al. [32].)

quencies and pressures that PWV was independent of frequency and dependent on pressure. On the other hand, Mangoni et al. [36] showed in anaesthetized rats that heart rate increases by pacing are accompanied by a reduction in local arterial distensibility, which is more pronounced in the elastic (carotid) than in the muscle (femoral) artery.

In contrast to the above studies, realised principally under 'passive' heart rate modification conditions which did not show significant variations of PWV with heart rate, more recent studies suggested some variable relationships between these two parameters under 'active' or normal conditions. We analysed in hypertensive patients the relationships between carotid-femoral PWV and blood pressure and heart rate using different methods and showed a significant relationship with the heart rate measured during daytime under ambulatory conditions *(figure 16)*; no similar results were observed with heart rate measured in clinic using casual methods or monitoring over 30 minutes *(table I)* [32]. Such association may be explained by the greater arterial degeneration caused by chronic elevation in heart rate (more fatiguing cycles).

Moreover, analysis of the results published by Girerd et al. [37] in borderline hypertension and by Pannier et al. [38] in established hypertension showed higher values of pulse wave velocities in hypertensive patients, and revealed also that hypertensives presented higher values of heart rate in comparison to normotensives. Despite this significant difference, the role of the heart rate in increasing PWV was not discussed in their respective analyses, probably because it was not previously described at that date. More recently, Sa Cunha et al. [39] analysed the association between high heart rate and high arterial rigidity in normotensive and hypertensive subjects. Their results showed that high heart rate was strongly associated with elevated PWV even after adjustment for age and blood pressure. These associations differed according to the arterial segment (significant associations were found for the aorta and the lower limbs but not for the arm) and sex (higher significant associations were observed in men) *(table II)*. In a com-

TABLE II. Robust multiple regression analysis of factors influencing PWV of the aorta (A), the leg (B) and the arm (C). (Adapted from Sa Cunha et al. [39].) Independent variables in the analysis were age, weight, height, systolic blood pressure (SBP), diastolic blood pressure (DBP), and heart rate.

A – Aorta

Variable	B	t	Probability	Added R^2
For men				
Age (years)	0.69	20.8	0.0001	0.36
SBP (mmHg)	0.41	13.1	0.0001	0.14
Heart rate (b/min)	0.15	5.0	0.0001	0.02
Height (cm)	0.07	.2	0.03	
$R^2 = 0.88$, $F = 265.37$, $p < 0.0001$				
For women				0.33
Age (years)	0.65	13.8	0.0001	0.03
SBP (mmHg)	0.29	4.0	0.0001	0.03
Heart rate (b/min)	0.13	3.0	0.004	0.02
DBP (mmHg)	0.15	2.2	0.03	0.01
$R^2 = 0.85$, $F = 122.94$, $p < 0.0001$				

B: Standardised regression coefficient; t, t statistic for testing $B = 0$ against the alternate $B < > 0$; R^2, multiple determination R squared.

B – Leg

Variable	B	t	Probability	Added R^2
For men				
SBP (mmHg)	0.54	6.5	0.0001	0.12
Height (cm)	0.34	4.5	0.0001	0.06
Age (years)	0.30	4.3	0.0001	0.06
Heart rate (b/min)	0.15	2.5	0.02	0.02
Weight (kg)	− 0.17	− 2.3	0.03	0.02
DBP (mmHg)	0.18	2.1	0.03	0.01
$R^2 = 0.70$, $F = 39.51$, $p < 0.001$				
For women				
Age (years)	0.54	6.0	0.0001	0.25
DBP (mmHg)	0.34	3.8	0.001	0.01
$R^2 = 0.53$, $F = 38.15$, $p < 0.001$				

C – Arm

Variable	B	t	Probability	Added R^2
For men				
SBP (mmHg)	0.54	6.5	0.0001	0.12
DBP (mmHg)	0.62	10.5	0.0001	0.34
Age (years)	0.31	5.2	0.0001	0.08
$R^2 = 0.62$, $F = 100.67$, $p < 0.001$				
For women				
DBP (mmHg)	0.37	4.0	0.0001	0.13
Age (years)	0.27	2.6	0.01	0.05
Height (cm)	− 0.22	− 2.2	0.03	0.04
$R^2 = 0.50$, $F = 17.70$, $p < 0.001$				

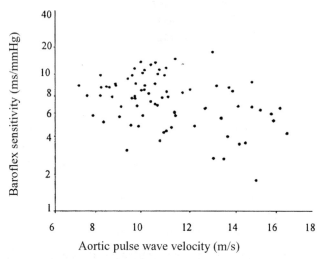

FIGURE 17. Relationship (on a logarithmic scale) between baroreflex sensitivity and aortic PWV. (Adapted from Sa Cunha et al. [39].)

plementary study, the same authors showed a significant inverse correlation between aortic PWV and the baroreflex sensitivity as evaluated from the relationship between systolic blood pressure and pulse intervals variations; high aortic PWV was associated with low baroreflex sensitivity *(figure 17)*. These results may be related to the frequency-dependent stress–strain relationship of the arterial wall under dynamic conditions.

Elsewhere, several studies analysing the determinants of PWV in normotensive, hypertensive and other populations according to the multiple regression analysis failed to show a constant relationship between PWV and heart rate, whereas others showed heart rate as a minor determinant of principally aortic pulse wave in some subgroups of the population. Recently, therefore, Morcet et al. [40] showed in normotensive and untreated hypertensive subjects a positive relationship between heart rate and carotid-femoral PWV in men, which persists after adjustment for age, systolic BP, glycemia, HDL cholesterol and body mass index. Stepwise analysis showed heart rate as the second determinant of PWV in normotensive ($r^2 = 6\%$), whereas it is the third determinant of PWV in hypertensive subjects ($r^2 = 2\%$). Moreover, recent analysis from the Complior® study showed that heart rate is a minor determinant of carotid-femoral PWV (1%) in untreated hypertensive patients (personal data); furthermore, separate analysis in men and women showed heart rate to be a significant minor determinant of carotid-femoral PWV only in women ($r^2 = 1\%$), the three major determinants of PWV being age, systolic BP and sex [13].

In summary, these observations taken together suggest that 'passive' heart rate variations in one specific individual may not influence PWV, whereas 'dynamic' heart rate variations may slightly modify PWV. Moreover, the influence of heart rate on PWV must be considered differently in individuals and in populations. In fact, to evaluate the association between heart rate and PWV, in the former, the effects of 'passive' or 'dynamic' heart rate changes can be evaluated, whereas in the latter, the influence of heart rate as a chronic cyclical stress is assessed. In order to clarify the relationship between arterial distensibility and heart rate and its pathophysiology, further specific studies in different populations are needed.

SALT INTAKE

Sodium intake may influence the cardiovascular hemodynamics independently of the blood pressure changes themselves. Animal experiments suggested that elevated sodium intake is associated with structural alterations in large arteries, and several mechanisms have been suggested: sodium modifies arterial smooth muscle tone through different mechanisms involving sodium-potassium pumps, calcium exchange, activation of the sympathetic nervous system and the action of natriuretic factors. Several clinical trials and epidemiological studies have analysed this complex relationship between sodium levels and viscoelastic properties of the arterial wall.

Ageing is associated with increased arterial stiffness, increased arterial pressure and a higher prevalence of hypertension. All are usually regarded as normal ageing phenomena and it is normally considered appropriate to adjust the normal range of arterial pressure and arterial stiffness for age. However, it is well known that in undeveloped societies with low dietary salt intake, arterial pressure rises to a lesser degree with increasing age and the prevalence of hypertension is markedly less than in western societies with regular salt intake. Therefore, to establish an adequate relationship between arterial stiffness and salt intake, it is important to demonstrate that the relationship between arterial stiffness and salt intake is independent of the relationship between stiffness and blood pressure for a given age range. Such relationships have been investigated in epidemiological studies performed both in China and Australia. In a comparative study performed in China, Avolio et al. measured PWV at three different arterial sites (aortic, arm and leg levels) together with arterial pressure in two groups of healthy subjects living either in a rural or urban community [8, 9]. Serum cholesterol levels were similar and low in each group, whereas the prevalence of both hypertension and salt intake was significantly higher in the urban community. In the rural population with low salt intake, PWV measured at the three sites was consistently lower and increased to a lesser degree with age by comparison to the urban population; this finding was observed even when subjects were compared at the same age and blood pressure levels. This showed that the higher rate of increasing arterial stiffness with age in the urban community was independent of blood pressure but related to the marked difference in dietary salt, suggesting therefore that salt intake has an independent effect on arterial tone and arterial wall properties contributing to increased arterial stiffness with age (figure 18).

In another cross-sectional study performed in Australia, the same authors [41] compared PWV measured at three different arterial sites (aortic, arm and leg levels) in normotensive subjects who voluntarily followed a low-salt diet (mean intake 44 mmol/d sodium) to those measured in a control group matched for age and mean blood pressure with a regular diet. For both samples, subjects were divided into three age subgroups: in subgroup 1 (aged 2–19 years), PWV was similar in the normal and low-salt groups; in subgroups 2 (20–44 years) and 3 (45–66 years), pulse wave velocities measured at the aortic, arm and leg levels were consistently lower in the low-salt group than in the con-

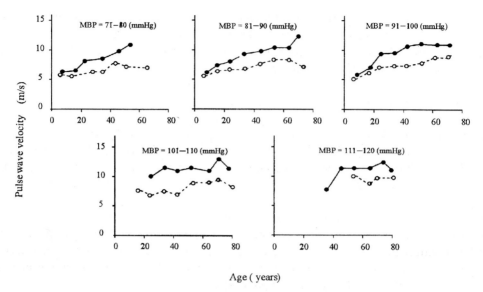

FIGURE 18. Relationships between aortic PWV and age in urban (●) and rural (○) Chinese populations at five levels of mean blood pressure (MBP). (Adapted from Avolio et al. [8].)

trols. These results suggest that normotensive adult subjects who followed a low-salt diet have reduced arterial stiffness and that this effect is independent of the blood pressure level *(figure 19)*.

Considering these findings and the results of Myers et al. [42], who showed that salt intake was associated with more pronounced increases of systolic rather than diastolic

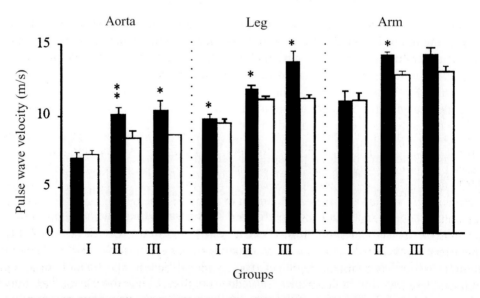

FIGURE 19. PWV at different arterial sites and in different age subgroups: I = 2 to 19 years; II = 29 to 44 years; III = 45 to 66 years in normotensive subjects following normal (■) or low-salt (□) diet. (Adapted from Avolio et al. [41].) * $p < 0.05$ ** $p < 0.01$.

blood pressure and to a greater extent in older than younger subjects, it seems likely that salt intake influences arterial stiffness in a manner that is independent of blood pressure, and that this influence is more pronounced in older than in younger subjects. Further support of this hypothesis was obtained by Levenson et al. [43], from their study of intravenous administration of isotonic saline (2 L in 120 minutes) to elderly subjects with systolic hypertension and arteriosclerosis obliterans of the lower limbs. Their results showed that isotonic saline caused a significant increase in systolic blood pressure with a decrease in the forearm arterial compliance. Similar observations were made by London et al. [44] in patients with severe hypertension and end-stage renal disease undergoing hemodialysis. Such patients are characterized by striking arterial damage involving calcifications and increased indices of arterial stiffness; aortic PWV was shown to be increased and associated with positive sodium balance, as assessed from interdialytic body-weight changes independent of age and blood pressure levels. The same authors showed that after antihypertensive treatment, changes of aortic PWV were poorly correlated with the blood pressure reduction and strongly associated with the interdialytic weight changes, thus indicating again the strong interactions between sodium balance and arterial stiffness in this particular population.

More recently, Draaijer et al. [45] studied arterial compliance at three different arterial sites: carotid, femoral and brachial in sodium-sensitive and sodium-resistant young male patients with borderline hypertension in comparison to age-matched normotensive controls. They showed that large artery compliance was significantly less in the sodium-sensistive than in the sodium-resistant subjects in all arteries studied. Compared with the controls, arterial compliance was reduced significantly in the sodium-sensitive group, whereas the sodium-resistant group did not differ significantly from the controls. For the authors, these results suggest alterations of the viscoelastic properties of the arterial walls in sodium-sensitive subjects with borderline hypertension.

Taken together, all these studies showed that sodium balance intake influences the geometry and stiffness of the arterial wall independent of age and blood pressure changes. Further studies are needed to clarify the mechanisms of the complex relationships between salt and the arterial wall viscoelastic properties.

GENETIC FACTORS

The genetic background may influence the large arteries in many ways. First, genetic disorders are responsible for some uncommon but severe monogenic cardiovascular diseases such as homozygous familial dyslipidaemia, Marfan's syndrome, Liddle's disease [46] and Gordon's syndrome [47]. Second, the association of several genetic and environmental factors leads to the development of many risk factors such as essential hypertension, dyslipidaemia, salt sensitivity and non-insulin-dependent diabetes [48, 49] responsible for arterial alterations. Finally, genetics can influence the vulnerability of the arterial wall to risk factors such as hypertension, ageing, cholesterol and smoking. In other words, for a similar degree of risk, arterial stiffening may be more or less pronounced as a function of genetic factors. Identification of such genetic markers may be of major interest in the detection of high-risk patients. In humans, some of these factors can now be identified by studying variants (polymorphisms) of genes coding for proteins that are implicated in cardiovascular regulation (candidate genes).

Nitric oxide synthase gene polymorphisms

Because of the important effect of nitric oxide (NO) on blood pressure, the arterial wall, and the reduced basal release of endothelial NO in hypertension, the gene of endothelial nitric oxide synthase (ENOS), which has been shown to be polymorphic [50], is a putative candidate gene for hypertension and arterial stiffening.

Studies focused on blood pressure revealed no linkage between hypertension and the ENOS gene [51]. More recently, Lacolley et al. [52] evaluated the association of arterial stiffness (PWV) with two recently described polymorphisms of the ENOS gene [51]; namely $G^{10}T$ polymorphism located in intron 23 ($G^{IN23}T$), and $G^{298}T$ polymorphism located in exon 7 ($Glu^{298}Asp$). They showed that the distributions of genotypes and allele prevalences of the endothelial nitric oxide synthase G^{10}-T polymorphisms among hypertensive and normotensive subjects were similar. In contrast, the prevalence of the nitric oxide synthase ^{298}G allele was higher in the hypertensive group than it was among normotensive subjects. No association of the endothelial nitric oxide synthase genotypes with blood pressure levels or PWV for either population was found (*table III*).

TABLE III. Multiple regression analysis of PWV on the endothelial nitric oxide synthase (ENOS) $Glu^{298}Asp$ and $G^{IN23}T$ and covariables. (Adapted from Lacolley et al. [52].)

Independent variable	Normotensive subjects		Hypertensive subjects	
	Partial R^2	Significance	Partial R^2	Significance
Age (years)	0.122	$p < 0.0001$	0.094	$p < 0.0001$
BMI (kg/m²)		NS	0.027	$p < 0.005$
SBP (mmHg)	0.084	$p < 0.0001$	0.138	$p < 0.0001$
Heart rate (mmHg)	0.022	$p < 0.04$		NS
ENOS $Glu^{298}Asp$		NS		NS
ENOS $G^{IN23}T$		NS		NS
Model R^2	0.241	$p < 0.0001$	0.255	$p < 0001$

Genetic factors of the renin-angiotensin system

Research interest is now focusing on the relationship between genetic factors of the renin-angiotensin system and modulation of large artery stiffness. The genes associated with this system have been studied for their effects on arterial disease [53, 54], and molecular biological techniques have been used to identify polymorphisms for several of these genes. Increasing evidence from human genetic studies now indicates that the ACE genotype is an independent risk factor for cardiac and arterial hypertrophy, and myocardial infarction [54], so that the renin-angiotensin system is directly implicated in these cardiovascular alterations. Most of the actions of this system are mediated by angiotensin II through stimulation of AT_1 receptors. The recent identification of AT_1-receptor gene A/C polymorphism thus suggests that the AT_1-receptors are involved in arterial alterations. This polymorphism is probably not functional but might be in linkage disequilibrium with an unidentified functional variant. It has been shown that the frequency of the AT_1C allele is increased in patients with severe hypertension or myocardial infarction [55].

Recently, polymorphisms of the renin-angiotensin system genes were evaluated for their effect on the development of aortic stiffness in hypertensive and normotensive subjects [56]. Arterial stiffness was assessed by measuring aortic PWV. The influence of angiotensin-converting enzyme gene polymorphisms (ACE – Insertion/Deletion – I/D) on aortic stiffness (carotid-femoral PWV) was evaluated by Benetos et al. [56] in normotensive and hypertensive patients. Their results showed that this polymorphism does not influence aortic stiffness in normotensives and that the ACE I allele is weakly associated to increased stiffness, with only an increasing trend of mean PWV values with the number of ACE I alleles (*table IV*). In contrast, Castellano et al. [57] have shown in the Vobarno study that increased medial-intimal thickness of the carotid artery is associated with the presence of the ACE D allele. These apparently conflicting results could suggest that the mechanisms involved in the development of arterial hypertrophy and stiffness are different. Indeed, it was shown recently that wall thickening of the large arteries is not necessarily associated with increased stiffness, indicating that other structural changes occur to regulate arterial elastic properties. However, we cannot draw clear conclusions about the influence of the ACE I/D gene polymorphisms on aortic stiffness; in fact, because of the low incidence of the II genotype, wider studies are needed to conclude this issue.

TABLE IV. Influence of ACE I/D genotypes on PWV in normotensive and hypertensive subjects. No difference between the PWV of the different genotype polymorphism groups was noticed. (Adapted from Benetos et al. [56].) Values are mean ± SD.

	Normotensive subjects				Hypertensive patients			
	II (*n* = 25)	ID (*n* = 56)	DD (*n* = 47)	*p* by ANOVA	II (*n* = 46)	ID (*n* = 159)	DD (*n* = 106)	*p* by ANOVA
Age	46.9 ± 10.0	42.4 ± 12.5	46.0 ± 9.8	NS	48.9 ± 10.2	49.0 ± 10.7	49.0 ± 10.7	NS
BMI (kg/m²)	24.5 ± 3.9	23.2 ± 3.5	25.0 ± 3.4	<.05*	25.6 ± 3.7	25.7 ± 3.6	26.0 ± 3.2	NS
SBP (mmHg)	122.0 ± 10.8	121.8 ± 10.1	125.5 ± 9.2	NS	153.66 ± 11.9	160.1 ± 14.4	155.6 ± 11.0	<.003*
DBP (mmHg)	75.6 ± 7.1	75.1 ± 7.6	77.6 ± 6.8	NS	93.5 ± 11.7	97.8 ± 10.5	94.5 ± 7.8	<.005*
PWV** (m/s)	9.1 ± 1.7	9.4 ± 1.9	9.0 ± 1.5	NS	13.1 ± 3.7	12.4 ± 3.2	12.0 ± 2.7	NS***

Values are mean ± SD. * Test of codominant effect, p = NS. ** ANOVA was performed on log PWV. *** Test of codominant effect, $p < .05$ after adjustment for SBP and DBP.

Elsewhere, assessment of the role of angiotensin II type 1 receptor ($AGTR_1$ ^{1116}C) gene polymorphisms on PWV in cross-sectional studies has shown that in normotensives the AGTR1 polymorphism is not associated with aortic stiffness. In hypertensives the presence of the AT_1C allele was associated with increased aortic stiffness in both sexes, independent of blood pressure levels; this polymorphism explained 11.6% of the variance in PWV. The results of these studies may be related to several interactions.

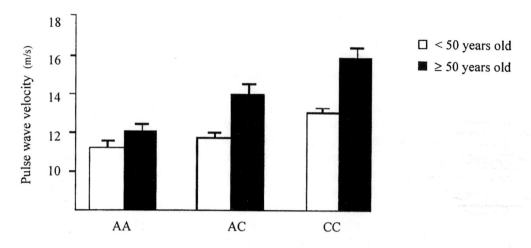

FIGURE 20. Influence of AGTR1 genotypes on PWV in hypertensive patients (adapted from Benetos et al. [58]). Association between angiotensin II AT$_1$-receptor genotype and aortic stiffness in both younger and older hypertensive patients; this effect is more pronounced in older patients. Patients with this mutation (presence of the C allele) develop, with age, more severe vascular stiffening than patients without the C allele, suggesting that this polymorphism could modify the effects of age on arterial stiffness.

First, the fact that AT$_1$ polymorphism is associated with aortic stiffness in hypertensives but not in normotensives may be related to a potentiation of the arterial effects of hypertension in some genotypes of the AT$_1$-receptor. This result is also consistent with experimental studies showing that angiotensin II-induced vascular smooth muscle proliferation in vitro was strongly enhanced by increased mechanical stretching, suggesting that hypertension-associated mechanical or structural alterations may be potentiated by angiotensin II receptor stimulation.

Second, the strong association between AT$_1$ genotype and aortic stiffness was observed in both younger and older hypertensive patients, but this effect was more pronounced in the older patients *(figure 20)*. In other words, older patients with the C allele (approximately 45% of the population) develop more severe vascular stiffening than patients without the C allele, suggesting that this polymorphism could modify the effects of age on arterial stiffness.

Third, an interaction was found between AT$_1$ genotype and the ratio of total cholesterol/high-density lipoprotein (HDL) cholesterol, affecting aortic stiffness. Thus in hypertensives presenting the C allele, a positive correlation was observed between this ratio and the PWV. In contrast, in patients without the C allele (AA homozygotes), an increase in the total/HDL cholesterol ratio was not associated with increased stiffness.

These results suggest that the AT$_1$ gene polymorphism is a particularly important risk marker for arterial stiffness, and could modulate the effects of hypertension, ageing and lipids on large arteries. Studies in larger populations are needed to corroborate these findings.

Role of the aldosterone synthase gene polymorphisms

The renin-angiotensin-aldosterone system plays an important role in large artery structure and blood pressure homeostasis. Among the genes coding for different components of this system, the aldosterone synthase (CYP11B2) gene could play an important role, but has been less investigated. The role of two variants of the aldosterone synthase gene (CYP11B2), one located in the promoter of the gene, $T^{-344}C$, the other in the 7th exon, the $T^{4896}C$ (Val/Ala), on plasma levels of renin and aldosterone, blood pressure and arterial stiffness, has been evaluated in subjects with essential hypertension by Pojoga et al. [59]. Their results showed that the presence of the ^{-344}C allele was associated with elevated levels of plasma aldosterone and PWV. No association was found between the $T^{4896}C$ polymorphism and the studied variables. Thus, in patients with essential hypertension, a common variant of the CYP11B2 aldosterone synthase gene, located on the promoter region, was found to be associated with significant differences in plasma aldosterone levels and arterial stiffness. These differences were not associated with variations in blood pressure levels *(table V)*.

TABLE V. Influence of aldosterone-synthase genotypes on PWV.
(Adapted from Pojoga et al. [59].) Mean values (SEM) of morphometric and hemodynamic variables according to the CYP11B2 $T^{-344}C$ and $T^{4986}C$ (Val^{386}Ala) polymorphisms.

	T^{-334} C				T^{4986} C		
	TT	TC	CC	ANOVA	TT	TC + CC*	ANOVA
Age	46.5 (1.4)	47.1 (1.1)	48.4 (1.7)	NS	46.9 (0.8)	48.3 (1.8)	NS
Height (cm)	170 (1)	171 (1)	170 (1)	NS	170 (1)	171 (2)	NS
Weight (kg)	74.6 (1.7)	74.9 (1.3)	75.3 (2.2)	NS	75.6 (1.0)	72.1 (2.2)	NS
SBP (mmHg)	150.1(2.3)	149.2 (1.8)	155.1 (2.9)	NS	150.8 (1.4)	152.0 (3.1)	NS
DBP (mmHg)	91.9 (1.5)	88.8 (1.2)	92.5 (1.9)	NS	90.1 (0.9)	92.0 (2.0)	NS
HR (bpm)	70.9 (1.5)	68.2 (1.2)	69.4 (1.9)	NS	69.3 (0.9)	69.2 (2.0)	NS
PWV (m/s)	11.3 (0.4)	12.7 (0.3)	12.0 (0.5)	0.022**	12.2 (0.2)	12.2 (0.5)	NS

* Due to the very small number, the ^{4986}C homozygotes ($n = 3$) were grouped with the TC heterozygotes.
** $p = .023$ after adjustment for age and systolic BP.

In summary, studies in normotensive and untreated hypertensive subjects on whether genotypes of the renin-angiotensin-aldosterone system (ACE, angiotensinogen, AngII AT_1 receptor, aldosterone synthase), endothelin (ETA and ETB receptors) and endothelial nitric oxide synthase may influence blood pressure levels and arterial stiffness have been performed recently. Benetos et al. [60] did not find any significant association between these genotypes and blood pressure levels. On the contrary, they found significant differences in aortic stiffness among the AT1 genotypes: in hypertensives but not in normotensives, the presence of the C allele of the Ang II AT1 receptor $A^{1166}C$ polymorphism was associated with increased aortic stiffness. Aldosterone synthase polymorphism (CYP11B^2 $T^{-344}C$) was also involved in arterial stiffness regulation.

Another important point is that human essential hypertension is a very multifactorial and heterogeneous disease and this heterogeneity influences the response to the antihypertensive drugs. Clinicians have very few markers indicating which mechanisms are predominant in each hypertensive. Such markers could have a major interest in thera-peutic strategies and drug choice. It has been suggested that plasma levels of renin or ACE could be helpful in determining the type of drug therapy for hypertension. Else-where, the same authors reported that AngII receptor AT1 A^{1166}C polymorphism influ-ences the effects of antihypertensive drugs on blood pressure and large arteries. Thus, in patients carrying the C allele, blood pressure reduction and regression of arterial stiff-ness were more pronounced with ACE inhibitors than with calcium antagonists, whereas the inverse tendency was observed in AA homozygotes [60]. These results, which need to be confirmed by wider studies, suggest that determination of genetic polymorphisms may be of interest in order to identify high-risk patients and to choose the type of anti-hypertensive therapy.

OTHERS

Respiration

Another factor that may modify the velocity of the pulse wave is respiration. Hickson et al. [61] showed that the velocity of the pulse wave varies with respiratory changes, being slightly higher during expiration than inspiration, owning to the fact that during the expiratory phase, the blood pressure is slightly increased. Thus, in order to obtain com-parable points for measurements in similar phases of respiration, a respiratory curve was recorded simultaneously with the pulse wave tracings. The observed differences of pulse wave velocities between the inspiratory and expiratory phases were less than 0.5 m/s (< 5%) in normal subjects (*figure 21*).

In order to consider the effect of respiration on PWV, measurements are usually per-formed on ten successive pulse waves or during ten seconds, which allows covering a complete respiratory cycle.

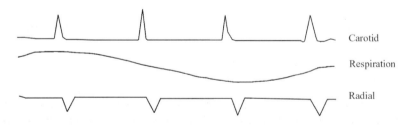

FIGURE 21. Recordings of pulse waves and respiration – carotid artery, respiration, radial artery.
(Adapted from Hickson et al. [61].)

Meals

Klip et al. [62] have analysed the influence of meals on PWV in young men. They noticed that after a meal there is a significant increase of PWV in peripheral vessels, whereas in the aorta a tendency toward decreasing PWV was noted. For the authors, the exact reason for this was not established, but one can theorize that immediately after a meal there is peripheral vasoconstriction with vasodilatation in the splanchnic area (*table VI*).

TABLE VI. PWV measurements before and after a meal. (Adapted from Klip et al. [62].)
(± 1 standard deviation)

PWV (m/s)					
Aorta		Leg		Arm	
Before meals	After meals	Before meals	After meals	Before meals	After meals
4.36 ± 1.3	4.23 ± 0.8	8.06 ± 1.0	10.28 ± 1.8	9.55 ± 2.3	14.60 ± 4.6

Blood flow

The blood flow velocity may affect in small amounts the PWV, hence it may be regarded as a small quantity in calculating the velocity of pulse waves. Assuming 0.75 m/s to be the average maximum velocity of the blood flow in the human aorta under basal conditions, and 0.25 m/s the average velocity in the carotid artery, it is obvious that the correction for the velocity of blood flow itself is small. But Bramwell and Hill [14] pointed out that any considerable increase in the velocity of the blood as a result of local or general disturbances will cause an equal increase in the velocity of the pulse wave. They stated that "any experimentally determined (pulse) wave velocity must represent the velocity of the wave relative to the blood, plus the velocity of the blood in the artery."

These observations may explain at least in part the increasing PWV observed in patients with 'hyperkinetic' hemodynamic or active tachycardia with increasing blood flow velocity.

Laboratory tests

Numerous studies have shown an increase of PWV during different laboratory sympathetic activation tests [63]. Effects of cold-pressor test had been described initially by Laubry et al. in 1921 [64] and reported later by a number of investigators in different populations.

Psychological stress tests, such as video games, reaction-time tasks, problem solving, etc., have been reported to increase arterial PWV as well as blood pressure and heart rate. Sympathetic activation and vasoconstriction have been described to underlie the observed increase in arterial stiffness [63].

For the same point of view, several authors reported the effects of neurovascular substances such as adrenaline, epinephrine, acetylcholine, etc., as an increase in PWV, with increasing vascular tone, BP, heart rate, etc., and corresponding decrease in vasodilation and blood pressure reduction [65].

Anthropometric factors

Numerous studies have analysed the relationships between arterial stiffness and several anthropometric parameters.

Chanudet et al. [66] analysed the determinants of carotid-femoral PWV in young male subjects; their results showed three parameters affecting PWV: 24-hour diastolic blood pressure, hematocrit and body surface area.

Toto-Moukouo et al. [67] studied brachial-radial PWV in obese and non-obese hypertensive patients. Their results showed a significant correlation between PWV and body mass index, a significant increase of PWV in obese patients independent of age, sex and blood pressure levels, and that body-weight reduction is associated with an improvement in arterial distensibility (*figures 22, 23*).

Giltay et al. [68] studied carotid and femoral artery stiffness with insulin sensitivity and body composition in healthy subjects. Their results showed that arterial distensibility is modulated by body composition in both men and women, but by insulin sensitivity

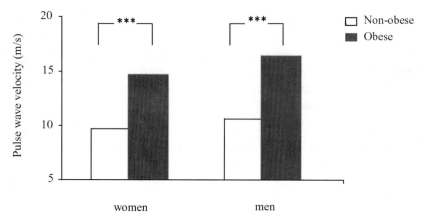

FIGURE 22. Brachial-radial PWV values in hypertensive obese and non-obese men and women. Differences are independent of age and blood pressure level. (Adapted from Toto-Moukouo et al. [67].)

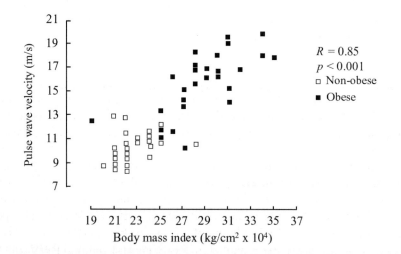

FIGURE 23. Relationship between body mass index and brachial-radial PWV in obese and non-obese hypertensive patients. (Adapted from Toto-Moukouo et al. [67].)

in women only; an independent association between insulin resistance and arterial stiffness was found to be more pronounced in women than in men. Elsewhere, Westerbacka et al. [69] analysed the effects of insulin on large-artery stiffness in obese and non-obese young men. Their results showed that insulin's effect of decreasing arterial stiffness in non-obese subjects is observed under physiological conditions and precedes a slow vasodilatory effect in the periphery; in obese subjects, insulin's normal effect is severely blunted. The degree of impairment of this vascular action of insulin is closely correlated with the degree of obesity.

The influence of body height on arterial hemodynamics has been investigated by London et al. [34, 70] in different populations. In normotensive and hypertensive subjects, body height is positively correlated with systolic pressure amplification from central to peripheral arteries and inversely correlated with the effect of wave reflections in central arteries. In patients with an end-stage renal disease and in control groups, no correlation was observed between body height and PWV measured at the aortic, upper-limb and lower-limb levels. In large populations including end-stage renal disease and normal renal function subjects, Smulyan et al. [71] found a significant relation between body height and carotid-femoral PWV.

Recently, we analysed the determinants of carotid-femoral PWV and its correlations with the anthropometric factors in the large hypertensive population of the Complior® study (personal data) [13]. The results showed significant correlations between aortic PWV and weight, height, waist circumference and waist/hip ratio. Analysis of the determinants of PWV showed age, systolic blood pressure, heart rate and height as determinants in the global population; only age and systolic blood pressure in men; and age, systolic blood pressure, heart rate, height and waist circumference in women [13].

In summary, anthropometric factors appear to be related to PWV in different manners according to the population analysed and the arterial site. In obese and non-obese hypertensives, PWV is correlated to body mass index; stiffness of the carotid and femoral arteries in healthy subjects seems to be modulated by body composition and insulin resistance; body height and waist circumference are related to the aortic PWV in hypertensives and end-stage renal disease.

Ethnic factors

Epidemiological studies have shown that the prevalence and severity of cardiovascular diseases are higher among those of African descent than Caucasians. Several hypotheses underlying this difference have been proposed; among these theories, Dustan in her 'keloid' hypothesis suggested that the excessive collagen production in blacks, as observed in keloid formation, may also be present in the vessel wall, resulting in changes in the vascular structure and function [72]. These racial differences in aortic stiffness in normotensive and hypertensive adults have been recently analysed by Ferreira et al. [73]. Carotid-femoral PWV was measured in normotensive and hypertensive policemen and soldiers who were classified as being of African or European descent. Their results showed that in the normotensive group, white subjects presented higher mean values of PWV than blacks, while the opposite behaviour was found in the hypertensive group (*figure 24*), differences which were even more significant after age adjustment. Moreo-

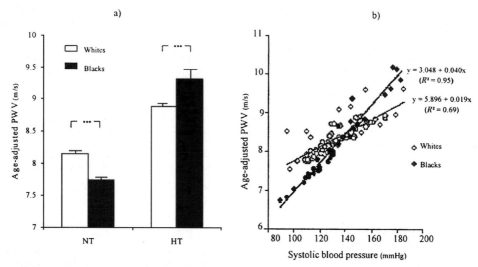

FIGURE 24. a. Comparison between age-adjusted PWV in white and black normotensives (NT) and hypertensives (HT). *** $p < 0.001$. b. Relationship between age-adjusted PWV and systolic BP in white and black adult male subjects. (Adapted from Ferreira et al. [73].)
Significant difference in slope of the regressions between groups was noticed.

ver, linear regression analysis for age-adjusted PWV and systolic blood pressure showed that the slope was significantly greater in blacks than in whites, thus suggesting a greater pressure-dependent increase in aortic stiffness in blacks than in whites *(figure 24)*. These differences in arterial stiffness between the racial groups need to be confirmed by longitudinal large-scale studies.

REFERENCES

1 Benetos A, Laurent S, Hoeks AP, Boutouyrie PH, Safar M. Arterial alterations with aging and high blood pressure. A noninvasive study of carotid and femoral arteries. Arterioscler Thromb 1993 ; 13 : 90-7.

2 Aschoff L. Lectures on pathology. New York: Paul B. Hoeber; 1924.

3 Zon L. Effects of age on artery [dissertation].University of Minnesota; 1932. Cited by Hallock PH. Arch Int Med 1934 ; 54 : 776.

4 Benetos A, Asmar R, Gautier S, Salvi P, Safar M. Heterogeneity of the arterial tree in essential hypertension: a noninvasive study of the terminal aorta and the common carotid artery. J Hum Hypertens 1994 ; 8 : 501-7.

5 Boutouyrie P, Laurent S, Benetos A, Girerd XJ, Hoeks AP, Safar ME. Opposing effects of ageing on distal and proximal large arteries in hypertensives. J Hypertens 1992 ; 10 Suppl 6 : 87-91.

6 Hallock P. Arterial elasticity in man in relation to age as evaluated by the pulse wave velocity method. Arch Int Med 1934 ; 54 : 770-98.

7 Laogun AA, Gosling RG. In vivo arterial compliance in man. Clin Phys Physiol Meas 1982 ; 3 : 201-12.

8 Avolio AP, Fa-Quan D, Wei-Qiang L, Yao-Fei L, Zhen-Dong H, Lian-Fen X, et al. Effects of aging on arterial distensibility in populations with high and low prevalence of hypertension: comparison between urban and rural communities in China. Circulation 1985 ; 71 : 202-10.

9 Avolio AP. Pulse wave velocity and hypertension. In: Safar ME, ed. Arterial and venous systems in essential hypertension. Martinus Nijhoff; 1987 ; p. 133-52.

10 Asmar R, Benetos A, Topouchian J, Laurent P, Pannier B, Brisac AM, et al. Assessment of arterial distensibility by automatic pulse wave velocity measurement. Validation and clinical application studies. Hypertension 1995 ; 26 : 485-90.

11 Asmar R, Benetos A, London G, Hugue C, Weiss Y, Topouchian J, et al. Aortic distensibility in normotensive, untreated and treated hypertensive patients. Blood Pressure 1995 ; 4 : 48-54.

12 Safar M. Arteries in clinical hypertension. New York: Lippincott-Raven; 1996.

13 Asmar R, Topouchian J, Pannier B, Rudnichi A, Safar M. Reversion of arterial abnormalities by long-term antihypertensive therapy in a large popu-

lation. The Complior® study. J Hypertens 1999 ; 17 Suppl 3 : S9.

14 Beyerholm O. Studies of the velocity of transmission of the pulse wave velocity in normal individuals. Acta Med Scand 1927 ; 67 : 203-35.

15 Schimmler W. A longitudinal study of the relationship between the pulse wave velocity in the aorta-iliaca vessel and the blood pressure. Basic Res Cardiol 1975 ; 70 : 46-57.

16 Smulyan H, Csermely TJ, Mookherjee S, Warner RA. Effect of age on arterial distensibility in asymptomatic humans. Arteriosclerosis 1983 ; 3 : 199-205.

17 Relf IRN, Lo CS, Myers KA, Wahlqvist ML. Risk factors for changes in aorto-iliac arterial compliance in healthy men. Arteriosclerosis 1986 ; 6 : 105-8.

18 Moens AI. Die Pulsecurve. Leiden, 1878.

19 Grunmach. Arch Fr Path Anat 1885 ; cii : 565.

20 Dawson. Proceedings of American Physiology Society. Am J Physiol 1917: xlii.

21 Bramwell JC, McDowall RJS, McSwiney BA. Proc Roy Soc 1924 ; 94.

22 Bramwell JC, Downing, Hill A. Heart 1923 ; 10 : 289.

23 Hickson SK, McSwiney BA. The effect of variations in blood-pressure on pulse wave velocity in the brachial artery in man. J Physiol 1924 ; 59 : 217-20.

24 Bazett HC, Dreyer NB. Measurements of pulse wave velocity. Am J Physiol 1922 ; 63 : 94-109.

25 Sands J. Studies in pulse wave velocity. III. Pulse wave velocity in pathological conditions. Am J Physiol 1924 ; 71 : 519.

26 Steele JM. Interpretation of arterial elasticity from measurements of pulse wave velocities. 1. Effect of pressure. Am Heart J 1937 ; 6 : 452-65.

27 Wiggers CJ. Physiology in health and disease. Philadephia: Lea and Febiger; 1934. Cited by Steele [26].

28 Frank O. Die Theorie der Pulswellen. Ztschr F Biol 1926 ; 85 : 91. Cited by Steele [26].

29 Haynes FW, Ellis LB, Weiss S. Pulse wave velocity and arterial elasticity in arterial hypertension, arteriosclerosis and related conditions. Blood Pressure 1936 ; 11 : 385-401.

30 Eliakim M, Sapoznikov D, Weinman J. Pulse wave velocity in healthy subjects and in patients with various disease states. Am Heart J 1971 ; 82 : 448-57.

31 Ho KL, Avolio AP, O'Rourke MF. Aortic pulse wave velocity, a non-invasive index of left ventricular afterload and aortic stiffening in an Australian community. Fed Proc 1983 ; 42 : 1128.

32 Asmar RG, Brunel PC, Pannier BM, Lacolley PJ, Safar ME. Arterial distensibility and ambulatory blood pressure monitoring in essential hypertension. Am J Cardiol 1988 ; 61 : 1066-70.

33 Sonesson B, Hansen F, Stale H, Lanne T. Compliance and diameter in the human abdominal aorta – The influence of age and sex. Eur J Vasc Surg 1993 ; 7 : 690-7.

34 London GM, Guerin AP, Pannier B, Marchais SJ, Stimpel M. Influence of sex on arterial hemodynamics and blood pressure. Role of body height. Hypertension 1995 ; 26 : 514-9.

35 Callaghan FJ, Babbs CF, Bourland JD, Geddes LA. The relationship between arterial pulse wave velocity and pulse frequency at different pressures. J Med Engl Technol 1984 ; 8 : 15-8.

36 Mangoni AA, Mircoli L, Giannattasio C, Ferrari AU, Mancia G. Heart rate-dependence of arterial distensibility in vivo. J Hypertens 1996 ; 14 : 897-901.

37 Girerd X, Chanudet X, Larroque P, Clement R, Laloux B, Safar M. Early arterial modifications in young patients with borderline hypertension. J Hypertens 1989 ; 7 Suppl 1 : 45-7.

38 Pannier BM, Safar ME, Laurent S, London GM. Indirect, noninvasive evaluation of pressure wave transmission in essential hypertension. Angiology 1989 ; 40 : 29-35.

39 Sa Cunha R, Pannier B, Benetos A, Siché JP, London GM, Mallion JM, et al. Association between high heart rate and high arterial rigidity in normotensive and hypertensive subjects. J Hypertens 1997 ; 15 : 1423-30.

40 Morcet JF, Guize L, Asmar R, Pannier B, Safar M, Benetos A. Influence of heart rate on large artery stiffness. Am J Hypertens 1999 ; 12 Suppl 4 : 174A.

41 Avolio AP, Clyde KM, Beard TC, Cooke HM, Ho KKL, O'Rourke MF. Improved arterial distensibility in normotensive subjects on a low salt diet. Arteriosclerosis 1986 ; 6 : 166-9.

42 Myers JB, Morgan TO. The effect of sodium intake on the blood pressure related to age and sex. Clin Exp Hypertens 1983 ; 5 : 99-118.

43 Levenson JA, Simon AC, Maarek BE, Gitelman GJ, Fiessinger JN, Safar ME. Regional compliance of brachial artery and saline infusion in patients with arteriosclerosis obliterans. Arteriosclerosis 1985 ; 5 : 80-7.

44 London GM, Marchais JS, Guérin AP, Métivier F, Safar ME, Fabiani F, et al. Salt and water retention and calcium blockade in uremia. Circulation 1990 ; 82 : 105-13.

45 Draaijer P, Kool MJ, Maessen JM, van Bortel LM, de Leuw PW, van Hoof JP, et al. Vascular distensibility and compliance in salt-sensitive and salt-resistant borderline hypertension. J Hypertens 1993 ; 11 : 1199-207.

46 Shimkets R, Warmock D, Bositis C, Nelson-Williams C, Hansson JH, Schambelan M, et al. Liddle's syndrome: heritable human hypertension caused by mutations in the beta subunit of the epithelial sodium channel. Cell 1994, 79 : 407-14.

47 Gordon R, Klemm S, Tunny T, Stowasser M. Gordon's syndrome: a sodium volume-dependent form of hypertension with a genetic basis. In: Laragh J, Brenner B, eds. Hypertension: pathophysiology, diagnosis and management. New York: Raven Press; 1995. p 2111-3.

48 Jeunemaître X, Soubrier F, Kotelevtsev YV, Lifton RP, Williams CS, Charru A, et al. Molecular basis of human hypertension: role of angiotensinogen. Cell 1992 ; 71 : 169-80.

49 Thomson G. Mapping disease genes: family based association studies. Am J Hum Genet 1995 ; 57 : 487-98.

50 Nadaud S, Bonnardeaux A, Lathrop GM, Soubrier F. Gene structure, polymorphism and mapping of

the human endothelial nitric oxide synthase gene. Biochem Biophys Res Commun 1994 ; 198 : 1027-33.

51 Bonnardeaux A, Nadaud S, Charru A, Jeunemaître X, Corvol P, Soubrier F. Lack of evidence of linkage of the endothelial cell nitric oxide synthase gene to essential hypertension. Circulation 1995 ; 91 : 96-102.

52 Lacolley P, Gautier S, Poirier O, Pannier B, Cambien F, Benetos A. Nitric oxide synthase gene polymorphisms, blood pressure and aortic stiffness in normotensive and hypertensive subjects. J Hypertens 1998 ; 16 : 31-5.

53 Cambien F, Alhenc-Gelas F, Herbeth B, Andre JL, Rakotovao R, Gonzales MF, et al. Familial resemblance of plasma angiotenin-converting enzyme level: the Nancy study. Am J Hum Genet 1988 ; 43 : 774-80.

54 Cambien F, Poirier O, Lecerf L, Evans A, Cambou JP, Arveiler D, et al. Deletion polymorphism in the gene for angiotensin-converting enzyme is a potent risk factor for myocardial infarction. Nature 1992 ; 359 : 641-4.

55 Tiret L, Bonnardeaux A, Poirier O, Ricard S, Marques-Vidal P, Evans A, et al. Synergistic effects of angiotensin-converting enzyme and angiotensin-II type 1 receptor gene polymorphisms on risk of myocardial infarction. Lancet 1994 ; 344 : 910-3.

56 Benetos A, Gautier S, Ricard S, Topouchian J, Asmar R, Poirier O, et al. Influence of angiotensin converting enzyme and angiotensin II type 1 receptor gene polymorphisms on aortic stiffness in normotensive and hypertensive patients. Circulation 1996 ; 94 : 698-703.

57 Castellano M, Muiesan ML, Rizzoni D, Beschi M, Pasini G, Cinelli A, et al. Angiotensin-converting enzyme I/D polymorphism and arterial wall thickness in general population: the Vobarno study. Circulation 1995 ; 91 : 2721-4.

58 Benetos A, Topouchian J, Ricard S, Gautier S, Bonnardeaux A, Asmar R, et al. Influence of angiotensin II type 1 receptor polymorphism on aortic stiffness in never-treated hypertensive patients. Hypertension 1995 ; 26 : 44-7.

59 Pojoga L, Gautier S, Blanc H, Guyene TT, Poirier O, Cambien F, et al. Genetic determination of plasma aldosterone levels in essential hypertension. Am J Hypertens 1998 ; 11 : 856-60.

60 Benetos A, Cambien F, Gautier S, Ricard S, Safar M, Laurent S, et al. Angiotensin II AT$_1$ receptor gene polymorphism influences the efficacy of chronic angiotensin converting enzyme inhibition on blood pressure and arterial stiffness in hypertensives. Hypertension 1996 ; 28 : 1081-4.

61 Hickson SK, McSwiney BA. Effect of respiratory movements on PWV. J Physiol 1924 ; 59 : 217.

62 Klip W. Difficulties in the measurement of pulse-wave velocity. Am Heart J 1958 ; 6 : 806-13.

63 Dutch J, Redman S. Psychological stress and arterial pulse transit time. NZ Med J 1983 ; 96 : 607-9.

64 Laubry C, Mougeot A, Giroux R. La vitesse de propagation de l'onde pulsatile artérielle. Arch Mal Cœur Vaiss 1921 ; 14 : 49, 97.

65 Kraner JC, Ogden E, McPherson RC. Immediate variations in pulse wave velocity caused by adrenalin in short, uniform parts of the arterial tree. Am J Physiol 1959 ; 197 : 432-6.

66 Chanudet X, Bauduceau B, Girerd X, Clement R, Celton H, Larroque P. The influence of anthropometric factors, hemorheologic parameters and the level of arterial pressure on PWV. J Mal Vasc 1989 ; 14 : 15-8.

67 Toto-Moukouo JJ, Achimastos A, Asmar R, Hughes CJ, Safar ME. Pulse wave velocity in patients with obesity and hypertension. Am Heart J 1986 ; 112 : 136-40.

68 Giltay EJ, Lambert J, Elbers JM, Gooren LJ, Asscheman H, Stehouwer CD. Arterial compliance and distensibility are modulated by body composition in both men and women but by insulin sensitivity only in women. Diabetologia 1999 ; 45 : 214-21.

69 Westerbacka J, Vehkavaara S, Bergholm R, Wilkinson I, Cockcroft J, Yki-Jarvinen H. Marked resistance of the ability of insulin to decrease arterial stiffness characterizes human obesity. Diabetes 1999 ; 48 : 821-7.

70 Blacher J, Demuth K, Guerin AP, Safar ME, Moatti N, London G. Influence of biochemical alterations on arterial stiffness in patients with end-stage renal disease. Arterioscler Thromb Vasc Biol 1998 ; 18 : 535-41.

71 Smulyan H, Marchais SJ, Pannier B, Guerin AP, Safar ME, London GM. Influence of body height on pulsatile arterial hemodynamic data. J Am Coll Cardiol 1998 ; 31 : 1103-9.

72 Dustan HP. Does keloid pathogenesis hold the key to understanding black/white differences in hypertension severity? Hypertension 1995 : 26 ; 858-62.

73 Ferreira AVL, Viana MC, Mill JG, Asmar RG, Sa Cunha R. Racial differences in aortic stiffness in normotensive and hypertensive adults. J Hypertens 1999 ; 17 : 631-7.

CHAPTER

Alterations of pulse wave velocity in clinical conditions

HYPERTENSION

(See also chapter III, section on Blood pressure.)

Several studies have described higher pulse wave velocities in hypertensive groups in comparison to normotensive groups. However, these results were reported at variable degrees in the different studies according to the arterial segment, the blood pressure used for subject classification, age normalisation, and drug therapy [1-3].

It is now well established that arterial abnormalities are observed in hypertensive humans even at an early stage of hypertensive disease. These abnormalities can be attributed not only to the stretching effect of elevated blood pressure, but also to intrinsic alterations of the arterial wall which could represent either adaptive structural and functional changes secondary to the chronic increase in arterial pressure, or primary abnormalities of the vessel wall [4].

Borderline and white-coat hypertension

Girerd et al. [5] compared aortic (carotid-femoral) and arm (brachial-radial) pulse wave velocities in young patients with borderline hypertension to an age-matched normotensive control group. Their results showed higher values of pulse wave velocities in the borderline hypertensives, significant correlations between mean blood pressure and pulse wave velocities, and that the corresponding regression lines between mean blood pressure and pulse wave velocities differed between the two groups *(table I)*. These data suggested that the higher pulse wave velocities noted in borderline patients are not solely due to the elevated pressure but also reflect arterial wall changes. Since PWV may be affected by heart rate, it is important to note here that the influence of this parameter, which differed between the two groups, was not considered in the analysis *(figure 1)*.

Recently, similar results were observed by Glen et al. [6], who investigated arterial stiffness in patients with white-coat or persistent hypertension in comparison to normotensive controls. Their results showed that the white-coat and persistently hypertensive

TABLE I. Pulse wave velocities in normotensive and borderline hypertensive subjects.
(Adapted from Girerd et al. [5].)

	Normotensives n = 60	Borderline hypertensives n = 63
Age (years)	21 ± 2	21 ± 2
Mean blood pressure (mmHg)	95 ± 8	105 ± 8***
Heart rate (beat/min)	71 ± 13	77 ± 5*
PWV (m/s) • carotid-femoral • brachial-radial	6.8 ± 0.7 10.7 ± 1.6	7.6 ± 0.8*** 12.0 ± 1.4***

± 1 Standard deviation; * $p < 0.05$; *** $p < 0.001$.

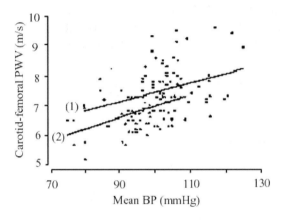

FIGURE 1. Correlation between PWV and mean BP in borderline hypertensives (1, ●) and normotensives (2, ▲). (Adapted from Girerd et al. [5].) For the same BP, the PWV is higher in hypertensives of the same age.

groups presented similar abnormalities of elasticity and stiffness *(table II)*. Elsewhere, Soma et al. [7] showed that blood pressure increase in subjects with white-coat hypertension is associated with increased peripheral vascular resistance and reduced arterial compliance. More recently, Lantelme et al. [8] showed that carotid-femoral PWV was increased in the hypertensives relative to the normotensives, even in the quartile of those with the lowest BP.

Established hypertension

Numerous studies have reported higher pulse wave velocities in patients with established hypertension. In fact, since the beginning of this century, several authors have described an increase of pulse wave velocities in patients with severe or malignant hypertension in case reports or studies performed on small groups of patients [2, 9-12]. More recently, different authors have reported similar results in mild to moderate essential hypertension [13-16]. Pannier et al. [17] compared aortic (carotid-femoral) and arm (brachial-radial)

TABLE II. Arterial changes in hypertension. (Adapted from Glen et al. [6].)

	Sustained hypertension	White-coat hypertension	Control group	ANOVA
Absolute distension (mm)	0.67*	0.67*	0.84	< 0.05
Distensibility (%)	11.4*	11.3*	15.0	< 0.005
Ep (kPa)	4.64*	4.36*	2.89	< 0.01
Stiffness index	4.53*	4.32*	3.27	< 0.05

* Significant difference compared with normotensive controls. Ep = elastic modulus.

pulse wave velocities in patients with essential hypertension to an age-matched normotensive control group. Their results showed: for the same age, higher values of pulse wave velocities in hypertensives; positive correlation of aortic PWV with age and with blood pressure; and brachial-radial PWV was not correlated with age, but with blood pressure to a lesser extent than in the aorta. These results suggest, at any given age, higher pulse wave velocities in hypertension principally in the aorta (table III).

TABLE III. Pulse wave velocities in normotensives and in patients with established hypertension. (Adapted from Pannier et al. [17].)

	Normotensives $n = 32$	Hypertensives $n = 91$
Age (years)	45 ± 2	44 ± 1
Mean blood pressure (mmHg)	93 ± 1	121 ± 1***
Heart rate (beat/min)	64 ± 1	74 ± 1***
PWV (m/s) • carotid-femoral • brachial-radial	 9.0 ± 0.3 8.9 ± 0.3	 10.6 ± 0.2*** 9.8 ± 0.2*

± 1 Standard deviation; * $p < 0.05$; *** $p < 0.001$.

In order to analyse the effects of blood pressure and age on PWV, the use of the product of age × blood pressure (diastolic) was proposed by Simon et al. [18], who studied hypertensive patients according to a nomogram obtained from normal subjects, relating this product to brachial-radial PWV. Their results showed that almost 70% of hypertensive values were inside the 95% confidence limits of the nomogram, suggesting that the increase of PWV could be related to the concomitant increase of blood pressure with age. However, about 30% of hypertensives were outside the nomogram with abnormally high brachial PWV when normalised for age and diastolic BP, thus indicating, according to the authors, the presence of early changes in the arterial wall. Using a similar approach, Armentano et al. [19] analysed the data according to a logarithmic model and showed that isobaric compliance (calculated using brachial-radial PWV) was decreased in hypertensives, thus confirming that reduced arterial distensibility and compliance of the brachial artery observed in hypertensive humans cannot be attributed solely to the stretching effect of elevated blood pressure [18, 19].

Elsewhere, in order to analyse the role of elevated blood pressure on the arterial distensibility reduction observed in hypertension, Gribbin et al. [13], then Smulyan et al. [16] used a pressurised box where the arm was placed and within which pressures can be changed positively or negatively, thus allowing measurements of the forearm pulse wave velocities at different transmural pressures. Their results in patients with systolodiastolic or systolic hypertension have shown that an increase in brachial-radial PWV with increased intra-arterial pressure could be abolished if comparisons were made at similar transmural pressure. According to the authors, these results suggest that increased arterial stiffness in the forearm is a consequence of the elevated distending pressures and not the cause of hypertension, thus not due to irreversible structural changes in the arterial wall. Nevertheless, these observations must be considered with caution because: 1) there was considerable scatter of the data; 2) the method offers data only on the forearm muscular arteries, but cannot be extrapolated to elastic arteries which are more important to consider in terms of stiffness and distensibility in hypertension and atherosclerosis; 3) both positive and negative box-pressures were assumed to be transmitted unchanged through the arm to the depth of the arterial wall, an assumption which may not be entirely true, particularly for negative pressures; and 4) measurements were made from relatively short distances and transit times. While these findings may be a combination of many factors, it is unclear how they relate to the central elastic arteries.

More recently, we analysed aortic PWV (carotid-femoral) in a large population of normotensive and hypertensive patients [1, 20] and showed higher PWV in hypertensives in comparison to normotensives (11.8 ± 2.7 versus 8.5 ± 1.5 m/s). Analysis of the correlations observed between age and PWV showed, at any given age, higher PWV in hypertensives with a significant difference between the corresponding regression lines (*figure 2*).

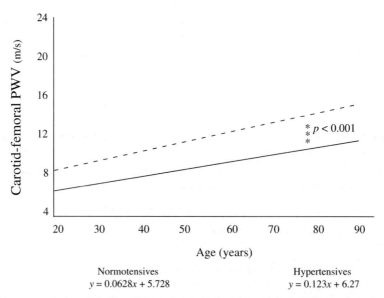

FIGURE 2. Linear correlations between PWV and age, in established hypertensive patients (----) and in normotensive subjects (—). The PWV is higher in hypertensives. (Adapted from Asmar et al. [1].)

In summary, taken together these findings showed:

– in borderline hypertension, higher carotid-femoral and brachial-radial PWV than in age-matched normotensives;

– in white-coat hypertension, increased carotid-femoral PWV and stiffness index, similar to those observed in sustained hypertension, by comparison to age-matched normotensives;

– in sustained hypertension, higher PWV of central arteries than in normotensives at any given age.

Elevated PWV and increased arterial stiffness cannot be attributed solely to the stretching effect of elevated blood pressure but also to early changes and abnormalities in the arterial wall in hypertension.

DIABETES

Diabetes constitutes one of the major cardiovascular risk factors. Atherosclerosis and arterial complications in diabetic patients appear to be progressively increasing and have been reported as the major causes of death in more than 50% of the fatalities in diabetic subjects. Therefore, several studies analysed the effect of diabetes on arterial stiffness and PWV and tried to determine whether these indices may be used as early indicators of the arterial wall changes observed in diabetic patients.

During the fifties, Lax et al. [21] analysed the alterations in the contour of the pressure wave as an index of atherosclerosis and vascular wall rigidity, and showed alteration in a high percentage of young diabetic subjects who had no clinical evidence of atherosclerosis and in 'normal' subjects with no evidence of diabetes but with a family history of diabetes. Later on, Woolam et al. [22] analysed the carotid-radial pulse wave in diabetic patients taking either oral hypoglycemic agents or insulin by comparison to healthy subjects; they reported higher PWV in diabetic patients even after considering age by using the value of the ratio between the observed PWV in diabetics and that predicted for the corresponding decade of age in healthy subjects. Moreover, higher PWV values were observed even in very young diabetic subjects *(figure 3)*. It should be noted here that the duration of the illness was not a precise measurement and that information on the degree of control obtained under the variety of therapeutic regimens was not available. The authors concluded that "high values of PWV were indicative of an incipient process of diffuse atherosclerosis and that the measurement of the PWV brought this into evidence earlier than the classic sign and symptoms. Serial measurements of PWV in diabetic subjects may permit early detection of atherosclerosis in these patients."

Since diabetes includes two major different entities of the disease, type 1 and type 2, which differ completely in terms of pathophysiology, and in order to better understand the relationships between arterial stiffness and diabetes, the authors considered each type of diabetes separately.

Diabetes – type 1

A number of studies have reported that type 1 diabetic patients have less distensible or stiffer arteries than normal subjects. However, most of these studies have not considered

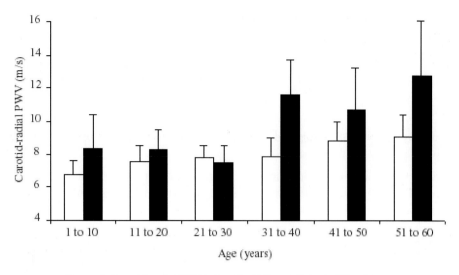

FIGURE 3. Carotid-radial PWV in healthy (□) and diabetic (■) subjects.
(Adapted from Woolam et al. [22].)

some important factors which may influence the results, such as the duration of the illness, the degree of obtained control under therapy, etc. (*table IV*). Stella et al. [23] showed higher PWV measured in the lower limbs of diabetic children with significant correlation between the elastic modulus and duration of diabetes. Christensen et al. [24] showed similar results for femoral stiffness in adults. Paillole et al. [25] showed higher aortic PWV in diabetic adults with good glycemic control and without previous microangiopathy or heart disease by comparison to healthy control subjects. Similar results were reported by Oxlund et al. [26] on aortic distensibility. Krause et al. [27] showed increased PWV in the lower limbs of diabetic adolescents and young adults, correlated to the diabetic duration. Okada et al. [28] reported that the increasing rate of the brachial PWV from the supine to upright position was related to autonomic neuropathy. Lehmann et al. [29] analysed the aortic compliance in recent onset child patients. Their results contradicted reports in the literature and showed that the young type 1 diabetic patients evaluated within one year of diagnosis have aortas ranging up to 78% more distensible than their sex- and age-matched non-diabetic controls. Kool et al [30] reported reduced arterial distensibility only at the femoral level but not at the carotid and brachial arteries in uncomplicated diabetic adults. Ryden et al. [31] reported increased aortic and carotid stiffness in diabetic women but not in diabetic men. Similar results were reported more recently by Ahlgren et al. [32], who showed in diabetic women a significant correlation between aortic stiffness and diabetic duration and autonomic dysfunction. More recently, Lambert et al. [33] showed that acute hyperglycaemia had no effect on the arterial wall properties, whereas an association between arterial stiffness and heart rate variability has been described by Jensen-Urstad et al. [34]. Nevertheless, when we consider all the data published on this subject, all but one of the studies showed a decrease of arterial distensibility in type 1 diabetic patients. These arterial abnormalities, which have been reported even in young patients, children and adolescents, seem to be

TABLE IV. Studies on arterial PWV and stiffness in type 1 diabetes.

Authors		Method	Artery	Patients	Results	Comments
Woolam [22]	1962	PWV	Carotid-radial	Type 1 – Type 2 treated diabetics	Higher PWV in diabetics as compared to healthy subjects	No precise evaluation of the duration of illness and of the degree of glycemic controls
Stella [23]	1984	PWV	Lower limb	Children	Increase in PWV	Significant correlation with the diabetic duration
Christensen [24]	1987	Stiffness ultra-sound	Femoral	Adults	Increased stiffness in diabetics as compared with controls	Significant correlation with the duration of diabetes
Paillole [25]	1989	PWV	Aorta	Adults	Increased PWV in diabetics as compared with controls	Patients were normo-tensives with good glycemic control
Oxlund [26]	1989	Specific device	Aorta	Adults	Reduction of distensibility	Significant correlation with the duration of diabetes Aortic samples
Krause [27]	1991	PWV	Lower limb	Young adults, Adolescents	Increase in PWV in diabetics as compared with controls	Significant correlation with the duration of diabetes
Okada [28]	1992	PWV	Upper limb	Adults	Increasing rate of PWV from supine to upright positions was related to autonomic neuro-pathy	Heart rate variation coefficient was also found to be related to autonomic neuropathy
Lehmann [29]	1992	PWV (normalized compliance)	Aorta	Recent onset patients (children)	More distensible aortas in diabetics than their age- and sex-matched controls	Diabetics presented a mean age of 10 years with a duration of diabetes of 6 months
Kool [30]	1995	PWV & local distensibility	Aorta Carotid, Femoral & Brachial arteries	Adults	No differences were observed for the carotid and brachial distensibility Decrease of femoral distensibility No difference in aortic PWV	Only distensibility of the femoral artery was reduced in uncomplicated IDDM patients
Ryden-Ahlgren [31]	1995	Stiffness ultra-sound	Aorta Carotid	Adults	Increased aortic and carotid stiffness in diabetic women but not in diabetic men	Influence of gender on aortic and carotid stiffness in IDDM patients
Lambert [33]	1997	Distensibility ultra-sound	Carotid	Adults	No changes in arterial distensibility after acute hyperglycaemia	Subjects were healthy normotensives

TABLE IV. (continued).

Authors		Method	Artery	Patients	Results	Comments
Ahlgren [32]	1999	Stiffness ultra-sound	Aorta	Adults	Significant correlation between aortic stiff-ness and diabetic dura-tion in women but not in men	Significant correlation between aortic stiff-ness and autonomic dysfunction
Jensen-Urstad [34]	1999	Stiffness ultra-sound	Carotid	Adults	Association between stiffness and heart rate variability	Patients with stiffer arteries had lower heart rate variability

more pronounced at the aortic and the lower limb levels with significant correlation with the duration of diabetes. Measurement of arterial distensibility in type 1 diabetic patients has been proposed for early diagnosis of macroangiopathy. The pathophysiological mechanisms involved in the association between arterial stiffness and type 1 diabetes remain unclear. More specific large-scale studies are still needed.

Diabetes – type 2

Numerous studies have analysed arterial stiffness or compliance in type 2 diabetic patients (table V). Scarpello et al. [35] evaluated PWV in both upper and lower limbs in a series of diabetic and control subjects classified into three different groups: a) diabetic subjects with peripheral neuropathy; b) subjects with uncomplicated diabetes; and c) control subjects. Their results showed that in the upper limbs, PWV was similar for all groups; by contrast, in the lower limbs PWV was increased in patients with healed or ulcerated feet compared with controls, uncomplicated diabetic subjects or diabetic sub-jects with peripheral neuropathy alone. They suggested that increased PWV results from an underlying diffuse atherosclerosis, which is not detectable clinically and is found to predominantly affect the lower limb arteries rather than the upper limb vessels. Relf et al. [36] measured PWV down the aorta and iliac arteries in 45 healthy men and reported no correlation between arterial compliance and the area under the glucose tolerance curve. Lo et al. [37] evaluated early changes in arteries in the legs of non-insulin depend-ent diabetes mellitus (NIDDM) men with no clinical evidence of peripheral artery dis-ease and showed lower arterial compliance in diabetics by comparison to non-diabetic control subjects. Wahlqvist et al. [38, 39] analysed the determinants of arterial wall com-pliance in NIDDM by measuring aorto-iliac compliance. Their results showed a decrease in compliance in patients with diabetes, negative correlations between compli-ance and free fatty acid and insulin levels, and that arterial compliance was best pre-dicted on the basis of age and area under the blood glucose curve. They suggested that noninvasive investigations of arteries may be useful in the evaluation of pre-sympto-matic stages of atherosclerosis in diabetes. Lehmann et al. [29] analysed the aortic com-pliance in type 2 diabetic patients using measurements of PWV; their results support findings by other groups and showed that type 2 diabetic patients have significantly stiffer aortas than their age- and sex-matched non-diabetic controls. Megnien et al. [40] studied the effects of NIDDM on the physical properties of the brachial artery in men. Their results showed in comparison to control subjects, lower measured and isobaric

TABLE V. Studies on arterial PWV and stiffness in type 2 diabetes.

Authors		Method	Artery	Patients	Results	Comments
Woolam [22]	1962	PWV	Carotid-radial	Type 1 – Type 2 treated diabetics	Higher PWV in diabetics as compared to healthy subjects	No precise evaluation of the duration of illness and of the degree of glycemic control
Scarpello [35]	1980	PWV	Upper limbs Lower limbs	– Controls – Diabetics with and without peripheral neuropathy	– Similar PWV in the upper limbs in the 3 groups – Increased PWV in the lower limb of patients with ulcerated feet	Different results in the upper and lower limbs
Wahlqvist [38, 39]	1984	Compliance ultrasound	Aorto-iliac	NIDDM Controls	Decrease in compliance in NIDDM patients	Negative correlations between free fatty acid and insulin levels Association with the area under the blood glucose curve
Relf [36]	1986	PWV	Aorto-iliac	Healthy men	No correlation between arterial compliance and the area under the glucose curve	Subjects were healthy men
Lo [37]	1986	PWV	Lower limb	NIDDM	Lower compliance in NIDDM patients	No evaluation of the duration of illness
Lehmann [29]	1992	PWV "normalized compliance"	Aorta	NIDDM	Increased stiffness in NIDDM as compared to their controls	No precise evaluation of the duration of diabetes
Megnien [40]	1992	PWV	Brachial	NIDDM	Diabetics had lower measured and isobaric compliance	Fasting glucose correlated negatively with arterial compliance
Amar [41]	1995	PWV	Carotid-femoral	Hypertensives with elevated waist/hip ratio	Higher PWV in diabetics and glucose intolerant patients	Positive correlation between PWV and fasting glucose
Tanokuchi [42]	1995	PWV	Aorta	NIDDM	Age, systolic BP, duration of disease and serum creatinine were correlated to PWV	Multiple regression analysis showed age and BP as explanatory variables of PWV
Hopkins [43]	1996	PWV	Aorta	Normal subjects with and without family history of NIDDM	Subjects with positive family history of NIDDM had less distensible aortas, higher fasting glucose and insulin levels	Multivariate regression analysis showed family history of NIDDM as the only independent predictor of arterial compliance
Emoto [44]	1998	Stiffness ultrasound	Carotid-femoral	NIDDM	– Higher stiffness index in both carotid and femoral arteries in NIDDM – Inverse correlation between stiffness and insulin sensitivity index as well as with age and duration of diabetes	Association between arterial stiffness and insulin resistance in NIDDM

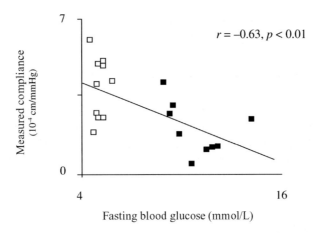

FIGURE 4. Correlation between measured and isobaric compliance and fasting blood glucose in the control (□) and diabetic (■) subjects. (Adapted from Megnien et al. [40].)

compliance (calculated on the basis of brachial-radial PWV) in diabetic patients. In the control and diabetic groups, fasting glucose correlated negatively with measured and isobaric compliance *(figure 4)*. Elsewhere, Amar et al. [41] studied the influence of glucose metabolism on carotid-femoral PWV in untreated hypertensive patients with elevated waist/hip ratio. Their results showed higher PWV values in diabetics and glucose intolerant patients in comparison to those with normal glucose levels; a positive correlation between PWV and fasting glycemia was noted *(figure 5)*.

More recently, Tanokuchi et al. [42] reported significant correlation between aortic PWV and duration of diabetes. Hopkins et al. [43] showed less distensible aortas in normal subjects with a positive family history of NIDDM. Moreover, Emoto et al. [44]

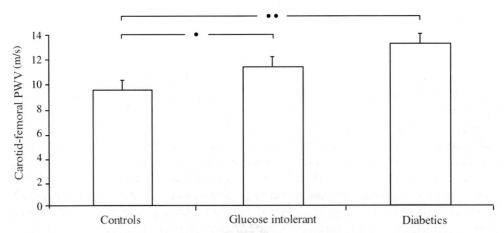

FIGURE 5. Carotid-femoral PWV in untreated hypertensives with elevated waist/hip ratio. (Adapted from Amar et al. [41].)

reported higher stiffness indices of both carotid and femoral arteries in NIDDM patients, with inverse correlation between stiffness and the insulin sensitivity index as well as with duration of diabetes.

Taken together, the published data showed higher PWV in NIDDM patients and also in normal subjects with a positive family history of NIDDM. Associations between PWV and fasting glucose and insulin levels as well as insulin resistance have been described. One study reported that these arterial abnormalities are more evident at the aortic and lower limb levels than in the upper limbs. More specific studies, taking into consideration the duration of the disease, its treatments and the degree of control obtained under treatment, are needed in order to understand the mechanisms involved between arterial stiffness and type 2 diabetes.

DYSLIPIDEMIA

Interest in arterial distensibility and dyslipidemia arises from animal experiments and clinical studies. Data from animals have shown an unexpected increase in aortic distensibility and compliance at an early stage of diet-induced experimental atherosclerosis, which subsequently fell (i.e., the aortas became stiffer) as atheroma progressed in the later stages of the disease [45, 46]. These findings have been partly confirmed by others who reported a decrease of aortic distensibility in animals exposed to grossly elevated plasma cholesterol levels with severe experimental atherosclerosis [47, 48]. In humans, increased serum cholesterol levels are known to be associated with increased propensity to coronary artery disease; similarly, increased arterial stiffness has also been associated with coronary disease [49-51]. However, increased cholesterol levels and altered arterial mechanical properties seem both to be associated with increased atherosclerotic disease. Moreover, several determinants of arterial distensibility, such as age, blood pressure level, etc., may also be associated with lipid metabolism and abnormalities. In fact, several authors have shown that hyperlipidaemia and hypertension co-exist more often than would be expected by chance, and epidemiological studies suggest that there is a positive relation between serum lipids and blood pressure. All these considerations highlight the difficulties in analysing the effect of isolated dyslipidemia on arterial distensibility and give explanations – at least in part – for apparently conflicting results concerning the effect of lipid metabolism on arterial stiffness (table VI).

Studies of Chinese [52] and German [53] populations failed to demonstrate any association between PWV and total plasma cholesterol. In these population studies, the different fractions of lipoproteins were not evaluated. Avolio et al. [54] found no significant correlation between PWV and serum cholesterol levels in patients with heterozygous familial hypercholesterolemia. Elsewhere, Lehmann et al. [55] investigated young patients (age < 24 years) with heterozygous familial hypercholesterolemia and matched normocholesterolemics on sex and age. They showed that patients with familial hypercholesterolemia had significantly more distensible aortas than the control subjects, with significant positive correlations between compliance and cholesterol, low-density lipoprotein cholesterol (LDL), duration of disease, and negative correlation between aortic compliance and high-density lipoprotein cholesterol (HDL). For the authors, these abnormal raised values of aortic compliance at the earliest phase of atherosclerosis (i.e., atherosis) are related to the infiltration of LDL-cholesterol into the intima and the formation of foam cells, which is likely to be the main event responsible for the initially raised aortic distensibility. Later, with advancing age, 'atherosis' develops a 'sclerotic' component due to laying down of connective tissue in the vessel wall, thus the arteries and the relationship between arterial distensibility and LDL-cholesterol will change [56] *(figure 6).*

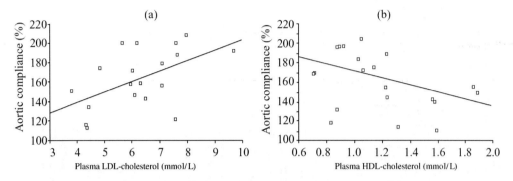

FIGURE 6. Correlation between aortic compliance (normalised for sex and age) and plasma LDL (a), and HDL cholesterol (b) levels in young patients with heterozygous familial hypercholesterolemia. (Adapted from Lehmann et al. [55].)

Moreover, the same authors [57, 58] analysed aortic distensibility in adults with heterozygous familial hypercholesterolemia and normocholesterolemics matched on sex and age. They showed that adults with familial hypercholesterolemia had significantly less distensible aortas than normocholesterolemics, with an inverse correlation between LDL-cholesterol and aortic distensibility in pooled data, age and LDL-cholesterol being the best independent predictors of aortic distensibility. Furthermore, similar significant inverse association between aortic distensibility and plasma LDL-cholesterol was reported in healthy adults [57, 58] *(figure 7).*

Relf et al. [59] studying healthy men, and London et al. [60, 61] studying patients with end-stage renal failure, found an inverse correlation between HDL-cholesterol and aortic PWV, while no correlation was found with total plasma cholesterol, as in the Chinese and German population studies [52, 53]. Pannier et al. [17], studying young subjects with borderline hypertension in comparison to normotensive controls of the same age, showed that about 25% of the borderline hypertensive patients presented significant dyslipidaemia. Only in this subgroup did subjects exhibit a strong positive relationship between aortic PWV and either plasma cholesterol or apolipoprotein B. There was no significant correlation between the lipoprotein parameters and PWV in the total population of borderline hypertensive subjects. Asmar et al. [1] showed no significant correlation between aortic PWV (adjusted for age and blood pressure level) and total cholesterol or HDL-cholesterol in untreated hypertensives, whereas a significant inverse correlation was observed between aortic PWV and HDL-cholesterol only in treated and well-controlled hypertensive subjects.

Dart et al. [62] reported that symptom-free adult patients with isolated hypercholesterolemia have more distensible aortas than normocholesterolemic controls, age and

TABLE VI. Effects of dyslipidemia on large arteries.

Authors	Population	Artery	Lipid metabolism	Results
Avolio [52]	Chinese population	Aorta	Total cholesterol	No correlation
Schimmler [53]	German population	Aorta	Total cholesterol	No correlation
Lehmann [55]	Young patients with heterozygous familial hypercholesterolemia – Controls	Aorta	Total cholesterol HDL – LDL	Aortic distensibility ↗ Positive correlation compliance / TC / LDL Negative correlation compliance / HDL
Avolio [54]	Adults with heterozygous familial hypercholesterolemia – Controls	Aorta Arm Leg	Total cholesterol	No correlation
Lehmann [55]	Adults with heterozygous familial hypercholesterolemia- Controls	Aorta	Total cholesterol HDL – LDL	Aortic distensibility ↗ Inverse correlation distensibility / LDL
Relf [59]	Healthy men	Aorta	Total cholesterol HDL	Positive correlation distensibility / HDL No correlation with TC
Kupari [65]	Healthy population	Aorta	Total cholesterol HDL	Inverse correlation stiffness / LDL
London [61]	End-stage renal failure	Aorta	Total cholesterol HDL	Positive correlation distensibility / HDL No correlation with TC
Pannier [17]	Young borderline hypertension – Controls	Aorta	Total cholesterol Lipoproteins fractions	No correlation in this population. Only hypertensives with dyslipidemia exhibit inverse correlation distensibility / TC / apolipoprotein B.
Asmar [1]	Normotensives – Untreated and treated hypertensives	Aorta	Total cholesterol HDL	No correlation in these populations Positive correlation distensibility / HDL only in treated patients with controlled BP subgroup
Dart [62]	Hypercholesterolemic symptom-free, coronary artery disease – Controls	Aorta	Total cholesterol LDL	Isolated hypercholesterolemia = distensibility ↗ Positive correlation distensibility / TC Steeper increase in stiffness with age in patients with coronary heart disease Inverse correlation stiffness / LDL in symptom-free patients

TABLE VI. (continued).

Authors	Population	Artery	Lipid metabolism	Results
Barenbrock [63]	Normotensive with hypercholesterolemia, without or with different degrees of CAD, treated hypertensives, controls	Carotid	Total cholesterol, HDL – LDL, Lipoprotein (a)	No correlation in normotensives. Distensibility ↘ in treated hypertensives and in hypercholesterolemics with 2 or 3 vessels CAD
Cameron [64]	Coronary artery disease, Controls	Aorta-Systemic	Total cholesterol, HDL – LDL	Stiffness index ↗ in CAD. Inverse correlation compliance / LDL
Moritani [66]	Healthy male volunteers	Arm	Total cholesterol, Triglyceride, HDL – LDL	Positive correlation between PWV and total cholesterol, triglyceride, as well as inverse correlation with HDL / TC
Giral [67]	Untreated hypercholesterolemic men	Aorta	Total cholesterol, HDL – HDL3, Triglyceride	Positive correlation between PWV and HDL, more specifically HDL3
Pitsavos [68]	Adults with heterozygous familial hypercholesterolemia	Aorta	Total cholesterol	Reduction of aortic distensibility without major modifications of aortic dimensions
Iannuzi [69]	Children with or without hyper-cholesterolemia	Aorta	Total cholesterol	No difference for aortic stiffness between the 2 groups. The slope of the regression equations (stiffness/age) was different between the 2 groups

cholesterol concentration being significant determinants of aortic distensibility index. They showed that patients with isolated hypercholesterolemia had a less steep increase in arterial stiffness with age than did their counterparts with normocholesterolemia. These apparently paradoxical findings were explained by the selection of patients with hypercholesterolemia who were symptom-free with no clinically evident atherosclerosis. The authors argued that these patients may be constitutionally resistant to the damaging effects of high cholesterol levels.

In a study of patients with coronary artery disease and raised cholesterol, the same authors demonstrated that the increase in aortic stiffness with age was more pronounced in hypercholesterolemic patients with coronary artery disease than in disease-free subjects, age and presence of coronary disease being significant determinants of aortic distensibility index *(figure 8)*. They suggested that aortic distensibility may be used as an indicator to distinguish between patients with and those without coronary artery disease.

Barenbrock et al. [63] analysed the effects of hypertension, atherosclerosis and hyperlipidaemia on the common carotid distensibility in normotensives and hypercholesterolemics without or with different degrees of coronary artery disease, treated hypertensives with no coronary disease and normocholesterolemia, and healthy controls matched for blood pressure level, sex and age. No significant correlation was found between carotid distensibility and cholesterol (total, HDL, LDL) or lipoprotein (a) levels in the normotensive patients. Carotid distensibility was lower in the treated hypertensive group (BP level not higher than in normotensives or controls) than in the controls, the group with no coronary disease and those with one-vessel coronary disease. Arterial distensibility was not lower in the hypertensives than in the group with two-or-three-vessel disease. These data showed that hypertension is a predominant factor in the development of reduced carotid distensibility. In hypercholesterolemic patients with coronary disease, the carotid distensibility is only affected in extended atherosclerosis (two or three vessels). For the authors, the extent of coronary artery disease is well correlated with the degree of atherosclerosis in the carotid arteries and they suggested that reduced carotid distensibility in normotensive hypercholesterolemics may be an indicator for severe atherosclerotic vessel wall changes.

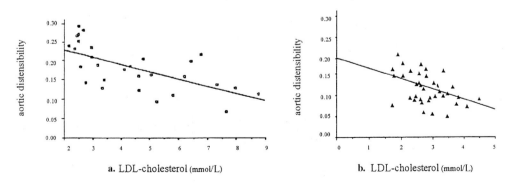

a. LDL-cholesterol (mmol/L)   b. LDL-cholesterol (mmol/L)

FIGURE 7. Relationships between aortic distensibility and LDL cholesterol levels in normocholesterolemic adults with heterozygous familial hypercholesterolemia (a) and in healthy adults (b). (Adapted from Lehmann et al. [57, 58].)

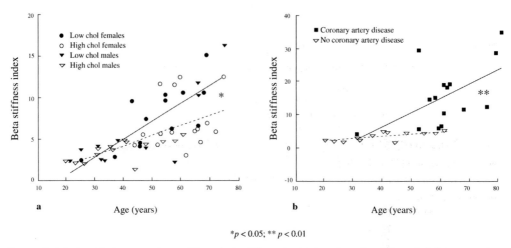

*p < 0.05; ** p < 0.01

FIGURE 8. Relationship between Beta stiffness index (dimensionless) and age in subjects free from coronary artery disease (a), and in hypercholesterolemic men with and without coronary artery disease (b). ——— low cholesterol; – – – high cholesterol. (Adapted from Dart et al. [62].)

Cameron et al. [64] analysed the relationship between arterial compliance, age, blood pressure and serum lipid levels in a group of newly diagnosed coronary artery disease patients and their controls matched for age, sex, smoking status and total serum cholesterol level. The Beta stiffness index was significantly higher in the coronary artery disease group (*figure 9*). Arterial compliance tended to decrease with an increasing plasma low-density lipoprotein cholesterol; for the groups combined, a significant negative correlation was demonstrated between compliance and low-density lipoprotein cholesterol; a nonsignificant trend towards increasing arterial compliance with an increasing plasma HDL level was noted (*figure 10*). Furthermore, a significant difference was found in the relationship between arterial compliance and diastolic blood pressure for the two groups; an inverse association between diastolic BP and arterial compliance being significant in only the coronary artery disease group. The latter finding suggests that compliance-pressure relationships differ between the disease and the disease-free groups.

Kupari et al. [65] reported in healthy subjects an inverse correlation between aortic elastic modulus and LDL cholesterol, and a positive correlation with HDL cholesterol.

Similar results were reported by Moritani et al. [66], who showed significant correlations between carotid-radial PWV and total cholesterol and triglycerides as well as inverse correlation with HDL/total cholesterol ratio in healthy male volunteers. Elsewhere, Giral et al. [67] reported that in untreated hypercholesterolemic men aortic PWV was related to HDL cholesterol and more specifically to HDL3 cholesterol subfraction; they suggested that HDL3 could have a prosclerotic stiffening effect. More recently, Pitsavos et al. [68] reported similar results to those of Lehmann et al. [55] in adults with heterozygous familial hypercholesterolemia, who exhibited significant reduction of aortic distensibility without major modifications of aortic dimensions. Finally, Iannuzi et al. [69] showed no difference for abdominal aortic stiffness in normocholesterolemic

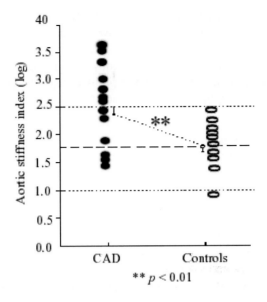

FIGURE 9. Aortic Beta stiffness index (log) between newly diagnosed coronary artery disease group (CAD) and matched controls. (Adapted from Cameron et al. [64].)

compared with hypercholesterolemic children, whereas the slope of the regression equations of stiffness versus age was different in the two groups.

In summary, numerous studies have evaluated the role of dyslipidaemia in arterial stiffness and distensibility in different populations *(table VI)*: general population, healthy subjects, normotensives, hypertensives, end-stage renal failure, coronary artery

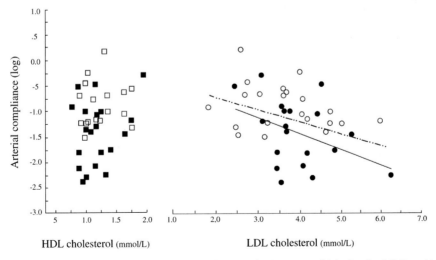

FIGURE 10. Systemic arterial compliance [log(SAC)] versus fasting serum high-density (HDL) and low-density (LDL) lipoprotein cholesterol levels for newly diagnosed coronary artery disease cases (■) and matched controls (□). (Adapted from Cameron et al. [64].)

disease, etc. Most of these studies have analysed the effect of lipids on the aorta, but very few have studied peripheral arteries such as those at the arm or leg levels. Whereas total cholesterol has been always evaluated, the other lipoprotein fractions have been analysed in disparate ways. Some of the results may appear inconsistent or paradoxical; however, these differences are likely to be explained largely in terms of major differences in methodology and subject selection. Nevertheless, some major points come to light from their results:

– in the general population and healthy subjects, no correlation was usually noted between arterial distensibility and total cholesterol; a positive correlation was observed with HDL cholesterol, and conflicting results have been reported with LDL cholesterol;

– in patients with heterozygous familial hypercholesterolemia, different results were observed; it seems that aortic distensibility increases at the earliest phase of the disease and decreases later with stiffened arteries;

– in hypertension, no correlation was observed between arterial distensibility and dyslipidaemia either in borderline or established hypertensive patients; correlations with total cholesterol, HDL cholesterol or apolipoprotein B were noted only in some subgroups;

– in patients with end-stage renal failure or coronary artery disease, a decrease in arterial distensibility was observed which mainly correlates with LDL (negatively) and HDL (positively) cholesterol levels.

Despite these observations, the role of lipid metabolism on arterial distensibility remains incompletely clarified and needs further investigations, which must also consider the effect of hypolipidaemic treatments.

ATHEROSCLEROSIS

(See also chapter VI on Pulse wave velocity and prognosis.)

Considering the complex relationships between atherosclerosis, age, blood pressure and the other cardiovascular risk factors which affect arterial stiffness, it appears very difficult to analyse the sole relationship between PWV and atherosclerosis per se.

Early in the 20th century, several authors noticed from descriptive studies or case reports the influence of atherosclerosis on PWV *(table VII)*. Conflicting results have been observed *(table VII)*. Friberger [70] first described in 1912 that carotid-radial PWV may be 'possibly' slightly increased in patients with arteriosclerosis, but not to a proportional degree with palpable thickening. Several authors [10, 11, 71] analysed PWV in individuals with perceptible sclerosis, with diagnoses of some of them verified by X-ray; their results in non-hypertensive patients with no complications of atherosclerosis showed that PWV in atherosclerosis without increased blood pressure is not higher than in individuals in the same age class without atherosclerosis. Conversely, other authors [9, 72-75] reported results with increased PWV in patients with arteriosclerosis without high blood pressure, and concluded that this certainly favours thickened vessels. Elsewhere, others [76-79] showed variable results in different patients or in different arterial sites (increased in central but not in peripheral arteries), which makes Sands [9] conclude, "In some instances the velocity of the pulse wave is increased and in others it decreased."

TABLE VII. PWV and arteriosclerosis
(descriptive studies and case reports published early in the 20th century).

Author	Year	Method	Arterial pathway	PWV observations
Friberger [70]	1912	Optical	Subclavian-radial	Possibly slightly increased. Not proportional to the palpable thickening
Ruschke [73]	1912	Optical	Carotid-radial	Increased
Münzer [74]	1912	Kymograph	Upper arm to calf	Increased in 1 of 3 cases
Silberman [77]	1913	Kymograph	Upper arm to calf	Variable
Laubry [78]	1921	Kymograph	Subclavian-radial Subclavian-femoral Femoral-tibial	Aortic may be increased Peripheral unaffected
Bazett [75]	1922	Polygraph	Apex-carotid Brachial-radial Femoral-dorsalis	Mostly increased
Bramwell [76]	1922	Sphygmograph	Carotid-radial	Theoretically increased
Sands [9]	1924	Optical	Apex-brachial Brachial-radial Apex-radial Apex-femoral Femoral-dorsalis	2 groups: • Increased in aorta but not in periphery • Increased in both central and periphery
Beyerholm [10]	1927	Modified EKG	Carotid-radial	Normal
Ude [79]	1933	Optical	Subclavian-femoral Femoral-radial	Increased in some cases
Turner [72]	1927	Optical	Carotid-radial	Variable
Eismayer [71]	1935	Optical	Arm, trunk, leg	Normal
Haynes [11]	1936	Optical	Subclavian-femoral Carotid-brachial Femoral-dorsalis	Normal

These conflicting reports may be related to numerous factors: 1) most of these studies were performed in a small number of subjects or were only case reports; 2) methods of measuring PWV and the studied arterial segments differ from one study to the other; and 3) no normalization or adjustment for the other determinants of PWV, such as age, blood pressure, etc., was performed. In order to consider these confusing factors and to avoid any misinterpretation, different approaches have been described.

Use of adjusted index

Considering that the major determinants of PWV are age and blood pressure, and in order to analyse the effect of arteriosclerosis per se on the arterial wall, several adjusted or normalized indices of PWV have been reported. Thus, Simon et al. [18] proposed the use of nomograms obtained from normal subjects relating PWV to the product of age and diastolic BP. According to their nomograms, they showed that in some hypertensive patients, arterial modifications may be related to the normal influence of age and blood pressure, whereas in other patients, an abnormally high PWV (outside the nomogram limits) reflected excessive arterial stiffness. Lehmann et al. [80] described a blood-pressure-independent index of aortic distensibility reported usually as being normalized for age and sex; they suggested this index to be a useful tool for assessing a patient's susceptibility to atheromatous arterial disease. Aortic compliance is deduced from the formula: $PWV^2 = K/r$, where r is the blood density and K the elastic modulus, and calculated per 10 mmHg pulse pressure as follows: $C = 66.7/PWV^2$. A compliance index (Ci), theoretically independent of blood pressure changes, is calculated using formula derived from a logarithmic elastic model: $Ci = C (\Delta P.10^3)/Ln(PS/PD)$, where PS and PD are systolic and diastolic BP and ΔP pulse pressure measured at the brachial artery. Whereas this latter approach has been used by other authors with different proposed distensibility or compliance indices, normalized for a given blood pressure level, further studies are needed to confirm the importance of its clinical application.

Criticisms raised against these types of adjusted or index-linked parameters are based on the concept itself. Indeed, if these normalization indices are interesting and correct in terms of mathematic modelization, their use in human clinic goes against medical logic. In fact, it is somewhat hazardous to extrapolate the evaluation of a hemodynamic parameter, measured in a specific patient under precise pathophysiological conditions, according to theoretical criteria issuing from another population or different conditions not fulfilled by that particular subject.

Comparative studies

Comparative studies between patients with atherosclerotic factors or lesions and their controls matched for sex and age showed frequently higher PWV or stiffness index values than those with or prone to atherosclerosis. Therefore, it has been shown that factors affecting arterial stiffness include those accelerating atherosclerosis such as hypertension, metabolic disorders, renal failure, etc., (see corresponding chapters). Moreover, studies of patients with atherosclerotic lesions showed increased PWV and arterial stiffness. In this regard, patients with end-stage renal disease have been described as showing an association between arterial hypertrophy and carotid distensibility, and between the presence of aortic calcification and the increase in aortic PWV [60, 61]. Nishio et al. [81] reported a significant correlation between aortic PWV and aortic calcification index in patients undergoing hemodialysis. Similar results were observed by Asai et al. [82] in elderly hemodialysis patients. In diabetic subjects, Scarpello et al. [35] showed increased PWV measured at the lower limbs in patients with healed or ulcerated feet, suggesting an underlying diffuse atherosclerosis. Jensen-Urstad et al. [34] reported in patients with type 1 diabetes mellitus a significant relationship between decreased heart rate variability and arterial wall stiffness. Taniwaki et al. [83] showed that the decrease in glomerular filtration rate in Japanese patients with type 2 diabetes is linked to atherosclerosis and carotid stiffness. In patients with hypercholesterolemia, Dart et al. [62] demonstrated that the increase in aortic stiffness with age was more pronounced in patients with coronary artery disease than in disease-free subjects. Barenbrock et al. [63] showed lower arterial distensibility in normotensive patients with two- or three-coronary vessel disease than in a control group with no coronary disease. For the authors, reduced carotid distensibility in normotensive hypercholesterolemics may be an indicator of severe atherosclerotic arterial wall changes. Cameron et al. [64] investigated a group of newly diagnosed coronary artery disease patients and found that arterial stiffness was higher in the coronary artery disease group. Lehmann et al. [80] showed an inverse relationship between atherosclerotic load (assessed by the number of cardiovascular risk factors and events) and aortic compliance in patients with vascular disease and/or diabetes. Blacher et al. [84] investigated elderly treated hypertensive patients and found that the presence of lower limb obliterans arteriopathy was positively correlated with carotid-femoral PWV.

Therefore, comparative studies performed in different populations showed that arterial stiffness or PWV are related to other atherosclerosis indices such as aortic calcification or to atherosclerosis vascular complications such as nephroangiosclerosis, coronary artery disease and atherosclerotic load.

Large-population studies

(See also chapter VI on PWV and prognosis.)

Analysis of arterial stiffness in large populations with different degrees of atherosclerosis have been performed by several authors.

To minimise the age-related effects of atherosclerosis on cardiovascular function, Avolio et al. [12, 52] conducted studies in Chinese populations with known low prevalence of atherosclerosis. The first study was conducted in urban Beijing and the second in a rural district. Their results showed that PWV increased with age in both groups but to a much greater degree in urban Beijing, where the prevalence of hypertension and dietary salt intake is higher.

Dart et al. [85] analysed the determinants of arterial stiffness in Chinese immigrants to Australia. Their results showed that regional aortic stiffness was significantly higher in the established immigrants compared with the recent immigrants. The increasing duration of Australian residence appeared to be accompanied by an increase in proximal arterial stiffness.

Namekata et al. [86] analysed the association between aortic PWV and atherosclerotic risk factors among Japanese Americans in Seattle, USA. They concluded that PWV may serve as a simple and valuable indicator to estimate the extent and severity of asymptomatic atherosclerosis in the large arteries.

Akisaka et al. [87] investigated the relationship between aortic PWV and atherogenic index in centenarians. Higher PWV was observed in centenarians than in the elderly group (70–89 years).

More recently, Van Popele et al. [88] investigated the association between indicators of atherosclerosis and PWV in the elderly population of the Rotterdam study. Their results showed (after adjustment for age, sex and blood pressure) that:

– cardiovascular risk factors that were significantly related to PWV were waist/hip ratio, HDL cholesterol, non-fasting glucose and prevalence of diabetes;

– indicators of atherosclerosis that were significantly related to PWV were: wall thickness of the carotid artery, ankle/brachial pressure index and aortic calcification. The results of this study in an elderly population show that arterial stiffness as measured by carotid-femoral PWV is related to cardiovascular risk factors as well as to indicators of atherosclerosis.

In summary, use of adjusted indices of arterial stiffness, comparative studies and large-population trials show that arterial stiffness and PWV are related to atherosclerosis risk factors, atherosclerotic lesions and complications, as well as to the other indicators of atherosclerosis.

CORONARY HEART DISEASE

Coronary heart disease (CHD) is thought to be associated with a generalized atherosclerosis process that begins in the large arteries. Since coronary artery perfusion occurs mainly during diastole, the elastic recoil of the aorta is necessary to produce the energy for the retrograde flow through the coronary arteries. More than ten studies have reported an association between elevated arterial stiffness and coronary heart disease.

Simonson et al. [89] first investigated normotensive men with coronary arterial disease (CAD) by comparison to healthy men in 1960. They showed, in comparable age groups, increased aortic PWV in patients with coronary disease in all age groups (≥ 40 years) with a mean difference of 1.68 m/s between patients with or without CAD (*figure 11*).

More recently, several populations with CAD have been investigated, usually by comparison to their controls without CAD: normotensives, hypertensives, hypercholesterolemics, diabetics, patients with myocardial infarction, etc., by different authors. The main methodological aspects and results of these studies are shown in *table VIII*. All of them but one (Eliakim et al. [2]) investigated the aortic and/or carotid arteries. Different methods including plethysmography, mechanical transducers, ultrasound and magnetic

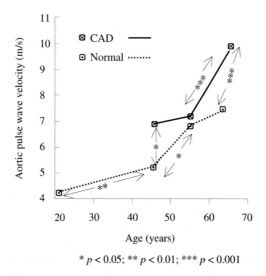

$* p < 0.05; ** p < 0.01; *** p < 0.001$

FIGURE 11. Increase in aortic PWV in normal subjects and in normotensive patients with coronary disease with age. Lines with asterisks show statistical significance between age groups. (Adapted from Simonson et al. [89].)

resonance were used to determine either PWV, Beta stiffness index or other distensibility indices. Most of their results showed an association between elevated PWV and arterial stiffness with CAD. Some of them reported altered arterial distensibility only in patients with extensive coronary atherosclerosis (two- or three-vessel disease), whereas others [90] showed proportional increase of arterial stiffness with the CAD severity (*figure 12*). In contrast, few studies showed no significant increase of arterial stiffness in patients with CAD, which gave rise to some comments. In the Eliakim et al. study [2], authors investigated the femoral-dorsalis arterial segment and not the aortic or the carotid artery as in the other studies. Megnien et al. investigated asymptomatic patients with cardiovascular risk factors and not patients with evident or symptomatic CAD.

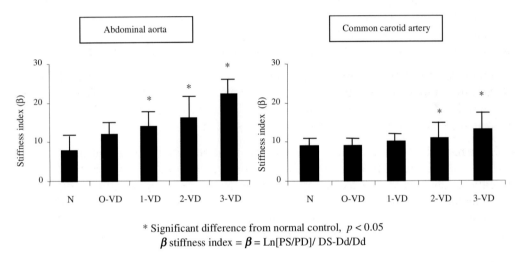

* Significant difference from normal control, $p < 0.05$
β stiffness index $= \beta = $ Ln[PS/PD]/ DS-Dd/Dd

FIGURE 12. Arterial stiffness index of abdominal aorta and common carotid artery in normal control group (N), patients with no significant coronary stenosis, (O-VD), and patients with 1-VD, 2-VD and 3-VD (vessel disease). (Adapted from Hirai et al. [90].)

In summary, several studies showed an association between elevated carotid or aortic arterial stiffness or PWV in patients with CAD. This altered arterial distensibility is more evident in patients with severe or high grade CAD than in asymptomatic patients or those with minor CAD.

CEREBROVASCULAR DISEASES

Theoretically, cerebrovascular diseases may be associated with either high or low levels of arterial stiffness, depending on the type of stroke, intracerebral haemorrhage or cerebral infarction. Abnormally low arterial stiffness may indicate a collagen deficiency and may be associated with ruptured cerebral aneurysms [97, 98]. In fact, studies based on arterial biopsies in patients undergoing surgery or on arterial samples obtained postmortem showed that deficiency of type III collagen was more frequent in patients with intracranial aneurysm than in their controls [97]. This deficiency has been described as being associated with an increase in the extensibility at stress values corresponding to

TABLE VIII. Studies of arterial stiffness and distensibility using noninvasive methods in patients with coronary heart disease.

Authors		Method	Artery	Patients	Results	Comments
Simonson [89]	1960	Plethysmo-graph	Aorta	Controls CAD	PWV ↗	Higher PWV in patients with CAD
Eliakim [2]	1971	Phethysmo-graph PWV	Femoral-dorsalis	CAD Heart failure	No difference compared to healthy subjects values	Similar PWV in nor-motensive with CAD and those without CAD
Bogren [91]	1980	Magnetic reso-nance/angio	Ascending aorta arch Abdominal aorta	Normal CAD	Compliance ↘	Decreased arterial compliance in CAD group
Hirai [90]	1989	Ultrasound β index	Abdominal aorta Carotid	Normal M.I.	β stiffness index ↗ in CAD	Stiffness index in aorta and carotid is higher in 3-vessel CAD and to a lesser degree in 1- and 2-vessel CAD
Dart [62]	1991	Ultrasound distensibility	Aortic arch	Normal hyper-cholesterol-emia. CAD car-diac transplant	Distensi-bility ↘	– Distensibility ↗ with age, steeper regres-sion slope in patients with CAD – Aortic distensibility = indicator of CAD
Ouchi [92]	1991	PWV	Aorta	Patients undergoing coronary angiography	PWV ↗ in 3-vessel CAD	Correlation between PWV and coronary angiography score but not after adjustment for age
Airaksinen [93]	1993	PWV	Aorta	Diabetes + CAD Controls + CAD	Higher PWV in the diabetic group	Collagen-linked fluo-rescence in the aorta and myocardium cor-related with PWV in diabetes
Trispos-kiadis [94]	1993	PWV	Aorta	NT with and without CAD	Distensibility ↘ in group with > 2-ves-sel CAD	High-grade CAD is associated with decreased distensibi-lity and PWV
Barenbrock [63]	1995	Ultrasound distensibility	Carotid	Controls NT + No CAD NT+ CAD HT + No CAD	Distensi-bility ↘ in HT and CAD with 2- and 3-vessel disease	Arterial distensibility is altered only in exten-sive atherosclerosis
Cameron [64]	1995	Ultrasound tonometry β index	Aorta Carotid	Controls CAD	β index ↗ in CAD Compliance ↘ in CAD	Systemic arterial compliance ↘ and β stiffness index ↗ in CAD

TABLE VIII. (continued).

Authors		Method	Artery	Patients	Results	Comments
Megnien [95]	1998	PWV Ultrafast tomography Ultrasonography	Aorta Coronary arteries	Asymptomatic + CV risk	No significant correlation after age adjustment	In symptomatic free subjects, aortic stiffness does not predict the presence of coronary and extra coronary atheroma
Gatzka [96]	1998	Ultrasound	Aorta	Previously unknown CAD Controls	Stiffness ↗ in CAD	– Higher aortic stiffness in CAD – Higher LVM index in CAD

blood pressure between 100 and 200 mmHg of the cerebral artery but not of the brachial artery [99, 100]. In contrast, other studies analysing the genetic risk factors for rupture of cerebral aneurysms showed that the frequencies of two polymorphic variations in the type III collagen gene may not differ in patients with cerebral aneurysm from their control, suggesting that atherosclerosis factors may contribute to the rupture of cerebral aneurysms [99, 100].

Alternatively, abnormally high arterial stiffness may indicate severe atherosclerosis and may be associated with cerebral infarction. Recently, Lehmann et al. [101] investigated aortic distensibility in patients with cerebrovascular disease on the basis of PWV measurements. Patients were studied at least seven days after their cerebrovascular events defined on the basis of computerized tomography to be in most cases as consecutive to cerebral infarcts. Their results showed that aortic compliance index was significantly reduced in patients with stroke compared with non-stroke age and sex-matched controls, corresponding to higher values for aortic PWV; moreover, stroke status was found to be a significant independent predictor of BP-corrected aortic distensibility (*figure 13*).

Elsewhere, owing to the fact that in hemiplegia there is decreased vascular tone on the paralyzed side, Haynes et al. [11] analysed the PWV on the two sides in five cases of hemiplegia. Measurements were performed at least ten days after the hemiplegia took

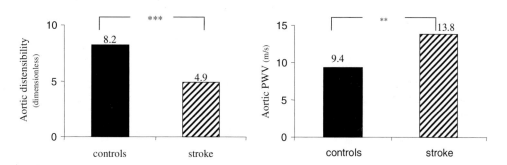

FIGURE 13. Aortic PWV and distensibility in stroke patients and control subjects. (Adapted from Lehmann et al. [101].)

place. The subclavian-femoral values on the two sides checked, as would be expected since the same vessel, the aorta, was chiefly involved, the velocities in the two arms and legs did not vary consistently. It is apparent that the PWV as measured in this study does not detect any tonus differences on the two sides *(table IX)*.

TABLE IX. PWV on the two sides in patients with hemiplegia.
(Adapted from Haynes et al. [11].)

	PWV (m/s)					
	Subclavian or Carotid-Femoral		Femoral Dorsalis-Pedis		Subclavian Carotid-Brachial	
Patients	Normal	Paralyzed	Normal	Paralyzed	Normal	Paralyzed
1	7.28	7.65	9.87	11.10	8.31	7.71
2	6.20	6.10	9.10	10.30	----	7.06
3	13.35	13.86	12.48	12.26	10.80	---
4	6.80	5.98	8.75	8.11	6.40	6.36
5	----	13.47	11.23	11.63	6.38	6.26

In summary, few studies have been performed to evaluate arterial stiffness in the different cerebrovascular diseases. Patients with strokes, mainly consecutive to cerebral infarcts, have been shown to present stiffer aortas. Specific studies are needed to understand the pathophysiological mechanisms of cerebrovascular diseases and to evaluate the predictive value of peripheral arterial stiffness in their occurrences.

HEART FAILURE

The importance of the peripheral vascular system is well recognized in cardiac heart failure (CHF), although many of the studies have concentrated on the small arteries, which are the predominant modifiers of peripheral vascular resistance and the steady afterload. Abnormalities in the large conduit vessels were demonstrated by several authors who showed, using invasive methods, that physical properties of the aortic wall are altered in patients with CHF. In fact, conduit artery distensibility affects the pulsatile component of the cardiac afterload and contributes to impaired left ventricular function. This may be partly reflected by the blood pressure reduction with heart failure, while PWV remains high. Fewer studies, using noninvasive methods, have been performed to evaluate the role of large arteries in CHF, and to determine whether comparable abnormalities to those seen at the ascending aorta are present in other parts of the arterial tree *(table X)*.

All but two of the performed studies showed that arterial compliance and distensibility evaluated at the aortic, carotid, iliac or brachial artery levels are impaired in different populations of patients with CHF *(table X)*. Arnold et al. [102] investigated patients with a broad range of clinical severity of CHF. Their results showed higher brachial PWV in CHF than in controls; this decrease of arterial distensibility and compliance became progressively lower as severity of CHF increased *(figure 14)*. Moreover, the authors

TABLE X. Studies of arterial stiffness and distensibility using noninvasive methods in patients with heart failure.

Authors		Method	Artery	Results	Comments
Eliakim [2]	1971	PWV	Femoral-dorsalis	Unchanged PWV	Unchanged or even slower PWV in CHF than in healthy age-matched subjects
Arnold [102]	1991	PWV	Brachial	PWV ↗	Compliance and PWV are progressively altered as severity of CHF increased
Lage [103]	1994	Ultrasound	Carotid	Distensibility ↘	Carotid distensibility was lower in CHF than in normals. Inverse correlations between distensibility and thickness, norepinephrine and aldosterone levels
Ramsey [104]	1995	PWV	Iliac	Distensibility ↘ by acetylcholine and increased blood flow in normal but not in CHF	– Effects of adenosine and trinitrate are preserved in CHF – EDRF mediated increase in distensibility is impaired in CHF
Giannattasio [105]	1995	Ultrasound	Radial	Severe CHF → reduction of compliance. No alteration in mild CHF Post-ischemic increase in compliance ↘	Arterial compliance and its modulation are impaired in CHF; more marked in severe CHF
Potocka-Plazak [106]	1998	PWV	Aorta	Similar PWV in elderly healthy and CHF subjects	– In very elderly subjects, no difference was observed between normal and CHF subjects – No significant correlation between PWV and norepinephrine, renin or aldosterone

noticed, while lower BP and flow in CHF might be expected to passively reduce distensibility which would be associated with a reduced PWV, the opposite was observed. These differences were probably not caused by underlying atherosclerosis alone, because patients with dilated cardiomyopathy and those with ischemic heart disease had similar changes in PWV. Thus, the observed changes in arterial properties may represent specific alterations associated with the pathophysiology of heart failure. Different causes of increased arterial stiffness in CHF may be involved: e.g., atherosclerosis, salt and water retention, stimulation of the sympathetic nervous system, the renin-angiotensin system, endothelium-derived vasoactive substances, the arterial natriuretic factor. In this regard, Lage et al. [103] investigated patients with congestive heart failure secondary to idiopathic dilated cardiomyopathy; their results showed that carotid artery distensibility was less in patients with CHF than in age-matched controls, and that carotid distensibility was inversely correlated with arterial wall thickness, plasma norepinephrine and aldosterone concentrations. Elsewhere, Ramsey et al. [104] investigated in

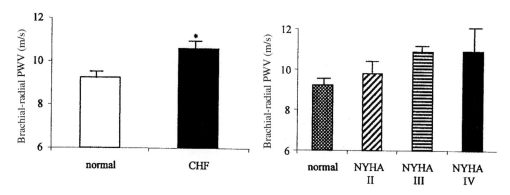

FIGURE 14. Brachial PWV in normal subjects and patients
with different degree of cardiac heart failure, NYHA. (Adapted from Arnold et al. [102].)

patients with CHF caused by dilated cardiomyopathy whether endothelium-mediated increase in distensibility is impaired in CHF. Their results showed that acetylcholine induced local reduction in PWV in healthy subjects but not in CHF, whereas adenosine induced similar reduction in PWV in both healthy subjects and CHF patients. Moreover, hyperhemic flow was associated with increases in distensibility in healthy subjects but not in CHF patients, whereas sublingual glyceryl trinitrate induced similar effects in both groups. These results highlighted the role of the endothelium on the arterial properties in CHF and implies that EDRF-mediated increases in distensibility are impaired in CHF patients. Concurrently, Giannattasio et al. [105] showed at the radial artery level that baseline compliance is altered in patients with severe congestive heart failure but not in those with mild CHF; however the post-ischemic increase in compliance was blunted in both mild and severe CHF, suggesting that arterial compliance and its modulation are impaired in congestive heart failure.

In contrast, Eliakim et al. [2] failed to find a significant difference of femoral-dorsalis PWV in patients with CHF by comparison to age-matched controls. This contrasting result may be related to the arterial site (lower limb) or to their CHF patients' characteristics since increase in PWV is accentuated with worsening severity of heart failure. More recently, Potocka-Plazak et al. [106] showed in very elderly women (82 years, 70 to 100 years) with congestive heart failure that aortic PWV in patients with CHF did not differ from figures in the age-matched healthy group. Their results suggest that age-associated arterial stiffening is a predominant factor in the development of reduced arterial distensibility in this particular population.

Hence, studies using noninvasive methods to evaluate the arterial mechanical properties of large arteries in CHF showed that aortic, carotid, iliac, brachial and radial distensibility or compliance are impaired in patients with dilated or ischemic CHF. These abnormalities have been noticed to be more pronounced in severe CHF and may be observed at baseline or revealed by hemodynamic tests. Different pathophysiological mechanisms of increased arterial stiffness in CHF may be involved. Further studies are needed to evaluate the role of arterial distensibility in the determination of the CHF prognosis and its improvement under treatment.

PERIPHERAL VASCULAR DISEASES

(See also section on Atherosclerosis, this chapter.)

Few studies investigated the effects of peripheral vascular diseases (PVD), namely obliterans arteriosclerosis of the lower limbs on PWV *(table XI)*. Principally, five studies

TABLE XI. Studies of arterial stiffness and distensibility using noninvasive methods in patients with peripheral vascular diseases.

Authors		Method	Artery	Results	Comments
Haynes [11]	1936	Optical PWV	Aorta Carotid-brachial, Femoral-dorsalis	PWV within the normal range values	– Only normotensive patients – No difference with controls of the same age
Simonson [108]	1955	Optical PWV	Heart – Feet Both legs	PWV ↘	– Only patients with PVD without hypertension – Recording of the toe pulse may slow the pulse transmission speed
Eliakim [2]	1971	Plethysmograph	Femoral-dorsalis	PWV ↘	PVD leads to a slowing of PWV in all age groups
Safar [107]	1987	Mechanical transducer	Brachial-radial	PWV within the normal range	– Brachial PWV in patients with arteriosclerosis obliterans of the lower limbs remains within the normal range – Reduced arterial compliance
Megnien [95]	1998	Mechanical transducer	Carotid-femoral	No significant PWV changes	– Number of extracoronary diseased sites is not associated to PWV – Lower PWV in patients with extracoronary and coronary lesions
Blacher [84]	1998	Mechanical transducer	Carotid-femoral	PWV correlates to lower limb obliterans arteriosclerosis	Significant correlation between PWV and arteriosclerosis obliterans of the lower limbs

investigated the association between PVD and PWV; their results are inconclusive. In fact, PWV was shown within the normal values by Haynes et al. [11], who investigated normotensive patients with PVD, and Safar et al. [107], who investigated the brachial artery. In contrast, lower PWV values in patients with PVD have been reported by Simonson et al. [108] and Eliakim et al. [2], who investigated PWV at the lower-limb level. Moreover, Megnien et al. [95] reported that the number of extracoronary diseased sites (carotid and femoral) is not associated to PWV, but their study included only asymptomatic patients with cardiovascular risk factors. When both extra coronary and coronary lesions are considered, lower carotid-femoral PWV values were observed in this sub-population *(figure 15)*. Elsewhere, Blacher et al. [84] recently reported obliterans arteriosclerosis of lower limbs as a significant determinant of carotid-femoral PWV in elderly hypertensive patients with arterial alterations.

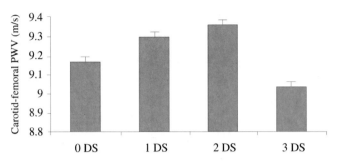

FIGURE 15. Carotid-femoral PWV values (adjusted for age) according to the number of extracoronary diseased sites (DS) in asymptomatic patients with cardiovascular risk factors. (Adapted from Megnien et al. [95].)

A combination of errors may lead to misinterpretation of the complex relationship between PVD and arterial stiffness or PWV. Thus, in order to limit some interference and to understand the pathophysiological mechanisms of this association, specific studies are needed.

Arterial stiffness in Marfan's syndrome

Several studies have described the arterial hemodynamic indices in Marfan's syndrome. Despite the greatly dilated aortic root, the aortic characteristic impedance has been reported in the normal range, suggesting increased aortic wall stiffness. Hirata et al. [109] measured the aortic stiffness index at the ascending and abdominal aorta with aortic PWV: their results showed decreased aortic distensibility, increased aortic stiffness indices in the ascending and abdominal aorta, with more rapid PWV in patients with Marfan's syndrome than in the normal subjects. Similar results were reported by Jeremy et al. [110], with greater aortic wall stiffness index and less aortic distensibility in the Marfan group than in controls. Elsewhere, Groenink et al. [111] reported using other techniques increased aortic PWV in Marfan's syndrome patients by comparison with control subjects. Recently, Jondeau et al. [112] showed that arterial distensibility was 38% lower in Marfan's syndrome than in control subjects at the site of the abdominal aorta but not at other sites: common carotid, common femoral and radial arteries. Therefore, these observations [113] showed that increased arterial stiffness and PWV are largely confined to the aorta, which is consistent with the histologic findings.

Arterial stiffness in Ehlers-Danlos syndrome

Few studies on arterial stiffness in patients with Ehlers-Danlos syndrome (EDS) are available. Matton et al. [114] reported that PWV was decreased in severely affected patients and normal in mildly affected subjects; lowered PWV reflected the increased arterial wall distensibility of affected patients. Similar results were observed by François et al. [115], who reported lowered PWV, indicating increased distensibility of the arterial wall in patients with Ehlers-Danlos syndrome. Elsewhere, recently Sonesson et al. [116] analysed the mechanical properties of the abdominal aorta and common carotid artery using ultrasound techniques in patients with different subtypes of Ehlers-Danlos syndrome. Their results showed that subjects with EDS had unaltered elastic modulus and stiffness indices in the aorta as well as in the common carotid; they suggested that the structural defect in the arterial wall collagen cannot be revealed under normal physiological conditions. Taken together, these observations emphasize the need of further studies to evaluate arterial stiffness in patients with EDS syndrome of different subtypes.

Arterial stiffness and aortic aneurysm

Several case reports have described altered PWV in patients with peripheral vascular diseases and namely in the presence of aortic aneurysm. In 1922, Bramwell and Hill [76] reported decreased carotid-radial PWV in patients with aortic aneurysm, whereas Beyerholm in 1927 [10] described scattered cases with no major significant changes of carotid-radial PWV. More recently, MacSweeney et al. [117] investigated the mechanical properties of the abdominal aorta in patients with aortic aneurysm and in patients with peripheral arterial disease. Their results showed that in the presence of a normal diameter, peripheral arterial disease had little effect on aortic stiffness, whereas aneurysmal dilatation was associated with a significant increase in aortic stiffness. Moreover, in patients undergoing aortic reconstruction, increasing aortic stiffness was associated with a decreased medial elastin content of the aortic biopsy. Vorp et al. [118] investigated the potential influence of intraluminal thrombus on the mechanical arterial properties in patients with aortic aneurysm containing intraluminal thrombus. Their results showed lower mean compliance for the abdominal aortic aneurysm wall alone than for the luminal surface enclosed by intraluminal thrombus. Boutouyrie et al. [119] investigated the mechanical properties of the common carotid artery and the abdominal aorta in patients with abdominal aortic aneurysm (AAA), and analysed the relationships between the viscoelastic properties and histologic lesions. Their results showed lower carotid distensibility in AAA patients than in hypertensive or normotensive subjects, lower distensibility of the aortic aneurysm than that of upstream aorta, itself being smaller than control aortas, even after adjustment for age and blood pressure *(figure 16)*. The mechanical properties of the arterial walls were not correlated with the grade of histologic lesions. Thus, data from case reports and clinical studies showed lower arterial distensibility in patients with AAA, observed at the carotid, carotid-radial and aortic levels.

RENAL FAILURE AND DIALYSIS

All the investigations performed at the beginning of this century have given the results that PWV, as a rule, is increased in the case of nephritis and chronic renal failure.

In 1912, Friberger [70] studied subclavian-radial pulse wave velocities in patients suffering from nephritis with palpable thickening arteries, using an optical device. His results showed an increase of PWV in patients with chronic nephritis (average = 11.8 m/s) by comparison to young controls (average = 8.2 m/s) attributed by the author to the higher muscular tension combined with degenerative changes in the arterial wall.

In 1912, Ruschke et al. [73] studied carotid-radial PWV in patients with nephritis, using an optical device; their results showed an increase of PWV in patients with nephritis (10-14 m/s, normal value = 9 m/s).

In 1922, the effect of nephritis chronica with hypertonia (hypertension) on carotid-radial PWV was evaluated by Beyerholm [10] using a modified EKG-based device. Their results

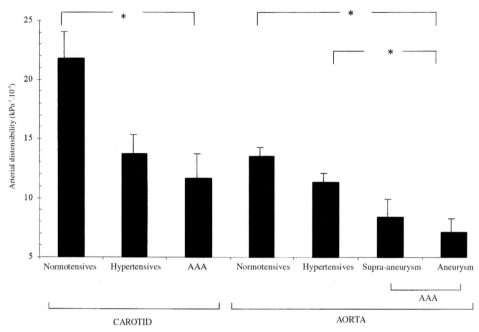

FIGURE 16. Arterial distensibility in patients with abdominal aortic aneurysm (AAA) in comparison with hypertensive and normotensive subjects. Values are adjusted for age, blood pressure and body surface area. (Adapted from Boutouyrie et al. [119].)

showed an average value of PWV for these patients of about 10.21 m/s, which is more than 3 m/s above the average of the normal values (7.13 m/s) and corresponds to an increase of about 50%. It will further be seen from their data that the increase in blood pressure and in PWV do not unconditionally accompany each other. They concluded that, "as a rule, PWV is increased in cases of nephritis chronica with hypertonia, but that blood pressure and PWV are not directly proportionate in their changes."

Eismayer et al. [71], in 1935, studied carotid-radial PWV in patients with chronic nephritis, uremia and nephroangiosclerosis and reported an average value over 10 m/s by comparison to normal values of 7.72 m/s.

Later on, several studies assessed arterial stiffness and PWV in renal failure and patients undergoing hemodialysis by comparison to control groups. They analysed the relationships between PWV and several clinical, biochemical and hemodynamic parameters, as well as their implications in terms of diagnosis and prognosis of cardiovascular complications. In this regard, London et al. [61, 120] analysed hemodialysis patients by comparison to controls of the same age and mean blood pressure and showed, in hemodialysis patients, higher PWV measured over the aorta (carotid-femoral) and to a lesser degree over the arm and the leg *(figure 17)*; significant correlation was noticed between the presence of aortic calcification and aortic PWV. Similar results for the aortic PWV and aortic calcification were observed by Nishio et al. [81] and Asai et al. [82].

Elsewhere, in order to analyse the role of PWV and wave reflections in the increased systolic and pulse pressures observed in patients with end-stage renal disease, London

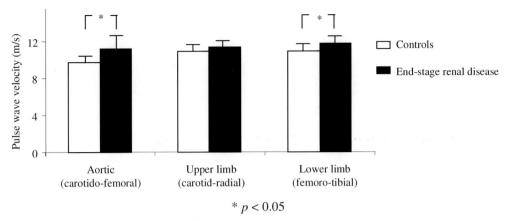

FIGURE 17. PWV in end-stage renal disease and controls matched for age, sex ratio and mean blood pressure. (Adapted from London et al. [120].)

et al. [120] showed, using pulse contour analysis, two principal factors associated with the increase in augmentation-index and shortened travel time of the reflected wave (determinants of the increased central pulse pressure). The first factor is the increased PWV, the second the smaller stature with shorter body height in dialysis patients. In another study [60], the same authors investigated the interactions between cardiac and arterial modifications in dialysis patients and reported parallel cardiac and arterial modifications with potential contribution of large artery alterations to the pathogenesis of left ventricular hypertrophy and functional alterations (*figure 18*).

Elsewhere, Amar et al. [121] observed in hemodialysis patients a positive correlation between aortic PWV and blood pressure variability as expressed by the diurnal variation coefficient and the ratio of nocturnal/diurnal blood pressure values assessed with 24-hour ambulatory monitoring. They suggested that an arterial distensibility impairment (as expressed by increased PWV) could enhance blood pressure variability and modify circadian blood pressure patterns.

Other studies investigated the determinants of PWV in end-stage renal disease. Demuth et al. [122] showed elevated plasma endothelin levels in end-stage renal disease patients, which was positively correlated to carotid-femoral (aortic) PWV. Blacher et al. [123] showed that carotid-femoral PWV was correlated to systolic blood pressure, age, prevalence of aortic calcification and prevalence of diabetes mellitus; carotid-radial PWV was influenced by mean blood pressure whereas femoral-tibial PWV was correlated to plasma total homocysteine and plasma endothelin. No independent correlation for any PWV was observed with cholesterol, HDL, triglyceride, fibrinogen or hemoglobin. Shoji et al. [124] showed in a hemodialysis population that VLDL, IDL and LDL cholesterol correlated positively with aortic PWV adjusted for age, gender, smoking and blood pressure, whereas Lp(a) did not; the authors suggested that aortic PWV in hemodialysis patients has a significant and independent association with IDL cholesterol, whereas in control subjects, it has an independent association with HDL cholesterol and Lp(a). Kishimoto et al. [125] investigated the correlations between PWV, plasma prostaglandins and lipids in dialysis. Their results showed that aortic PWV correlated with

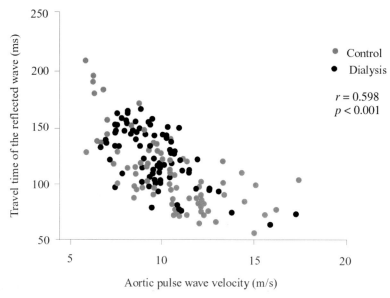

FIGURE 18. Correlation between aortic PWV and travel time of the reflected wave in dialysis patients and controls. (Adapted from London et al. [120].)

the plasma thromboxane A2 level. No significant correlation was observed between aortic PWV and the lipid abnormalities.

The prognostic value of carotid arterial stiffness as a predictor of cardiovascular and all-cause mortality in end-stage renal disease has been investigated by Blacher et al. [126]. Their results based on Cox analysis showed two dominant factors as predictors of all-cause and cardiovascular mortality: increased carotid arterial stiffness (incremental modulus of elasticity Einc) and decreased diastolic blood pressure. Lipid abnormalities and the presence of previous cardiovascular events interfered to a lesser extent.

In summary, all the case report publications and the clinical studies performed in patients with renal failure, end-stage renal disease and dialysis show an increase of PWV at the aorta, lower-limb and to a lesser degree at the upper-limb levels. This increase of PWV is independent of age, gender and blood pressure values. A parallel between the cardiac and arterial abnormalities has been reported. The correlation between PWV and the lipid metabolism parameters is variable. Significant correlations between PWV and the plasma total homocysteine, endothelin and prostaglandins have been described. Carotid arterial stiffness (Einc) has been shown as an independent predictor factor of cardiovascular and all-cause mortality in end-stage renal disease populations.

OTHERS

Arrhythmias

Eliakim et al. [2] analysed the effect of cardiac arrhythmias on the femoral-pedis PWV by beat-to-beat measurements made on 40 to 50 cardiac cycles in patients with atrial

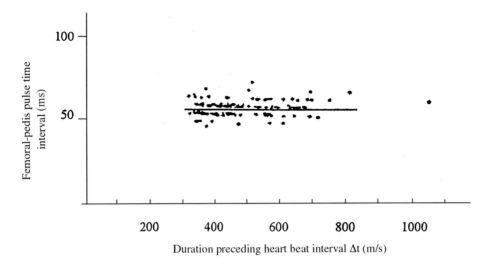

FIGURE 19. Relationship between the duration of the preceding heart beat interval and PWV in a case with atrial fibrillation. (Adapted from Eliakim [2].) Note that there was no change in velocity.

fibrillation. In addition, PWV generated by premature beats was examined by comparative measurements for premature and sinus beats in other patients with ventricular or supraventricular premature beats. Their results showed that in patients with atrial fibrillation, the PWV did not change significantly in spite of the large random variation in cardiac cycle length (*figure 19*).

In patients with premature beats, the results observed on a limited number of subjects showed that supraventricular premature beats generated a more rapid PWV than sinus beats (time interval = 80 m/s versus 102 m/s, respectively). On the other hand, in two other cases, the PWV of ventricular premature beats did not differ from that of the sinus and post-premature beats (*figure 20*). The authors concluded that with premature beats, "the propagation time of the pulse wave was unchanged in ventricular premature beats, or even increased in supraventricular premature beats."

Beyerholm et al. [10] analysed the effect of arrhythmia on carotid-radial PWV. In patients with arrhythmia perpetua, their results showed that the velocity of the pulse wave varied considerably, but showed no pronounced pathological values. Elsewhere, the same authors analysed the relationship between the velocity of transmission of the large and small pulse waves in patients with arrhythmia perpetua; no difference could be established between the velocity of large and small pulse waves.

It is important to note that the conclusions of the studies mentioned above were based on a limited number of patients or case reports and that some methodological criticisms may be argued. Hence, adequate studies are still needed to clarify the effects of cardiac arrhythmias and conduction abnormalities on PWV.

Growth hormone

Although vascular morbidity and mortality are increased in hypopituitary adults, there are limited data on the atherosclerotic process in these patients. Markussis et al. [127]

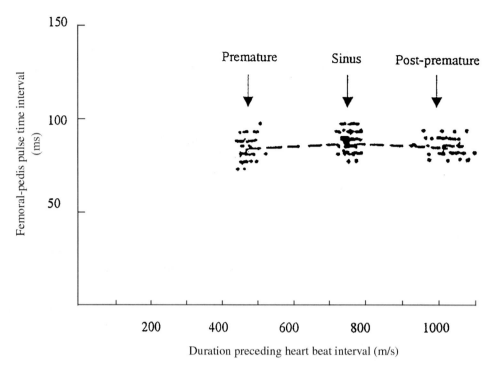

FIGURE 20. PWV generated by premature ventricular beats (left), sinus beats (middle), and post-premature beats (right). (Adapted from Eliakim [2].) Note that T remains constant for all beats.

reported an increase in carotid artery intima-media thickness in symptom-free hypopituitary patients on routine hormone replacement therapy. In another study, the same authors [128] showed asymptomatic hypopituitary adults (especially women) on conventional replacement therapy to have a lower distensibility coefficient and a higher β stiffness index of the common carotid arteries. Elsewhere, Lehmann et al. [129] showed that symptom-free growth hormone deficient adults have significantly less distensible aortas by comparison to a control group. Evidence for these observations comes from experimental studies which have shown that administration of biosynthetic growth hormone leads to changes in the concentration of elastin and type I collagen in the aorta, with an increase in aortic distensibility. Moreover, recently Pfeifer et al. [130] showed that growth hormone treatment of hypopituitary men reverses early morphological and functional atherosclerotic changes in major arteries; they suggested that growth hormone acts via insulin-like growth factor I, which is known to have important effects on the arterial wall.

Smoking

The effect of smoking on arterial hemodynamics has been evaluated in numerous studies including: healthy nonsmokers, healthy smokers, smokers and nonsmokers with other cardiovascular risk factors. The effect of cigarette smoking in healthy nonsmokers on the forearm arterial hemodynamics showed an increase of blood pressure, heart rate and PWV; these acute vascular effects of cigarette smoking were not prevented by a pretreatment with beta-blockers [131]. The effect of smoking on forearm haemodynamics in healthy smokers (10–15 cigarettes / 10 years) showed a significant increase in blood pressure, heart rate and PWV, a decrease in forearm blood flow and unchanged vascular resistance. This increase in PWV (+28%) was transient and peaked 15 minutes after smoking [132]. Failla et al. [133] investigated the effects of cigarette smoking in healthy smokers; they showed that radial artery distensibility was reduced only after smoking (– 41%), while carotid artery distensibility was reduced both during (– 33%) and after smoking (– 27%) versus before smoking. They concluded that acute cigarette smoking reduces distensibility not only in medium-sized but also in large elastic arteries, therefore causing systemic artery stiffening. Levenson et al. [134] analysed the effects of cigarette smoking on hemorheological variables (blood viscosity, plasma viscosity, microhematocrit) and on PWV in normotensive and hypertensive smokers and non-smokers. Their results showed that cigarette smoking and hypertension were independently associated with higher blood and plasma viscosity, hematocrit and PWV. Moreover, Nakamoto et al. [135] measured aortic PWV in adult cases of various arteriosclerotic diseases and showed that smoking was associated with increasing PWV levels and that "PWV was valuable as an index of arteriosclerosis... ."

In summary, numerous studies showed that smoking causes significant increase of PWV and arterial stiffness in both the medium-sized and large arteries.

Thyroid dysfunction

Cardiovascular manifestations are a frequent finding in hyperthyroid and hypothyroid states. Potential mechanisms by which thyroid hormones may exert their cardiovascular effects and pathophysiological consequences have emerged [9, 10, 136]. There is increasing evidence that thyroid hormones have a direct effect on the myocardium and the vessel walls and that they interact with the sympathetic nervous system by modulating adrenergic receptor function and/or density [137, 138]. Moreover, the serum level of type IV collagen has been described as closely related to thyroid hormone levels in patients with various thyroid diseases [139]. Pathophysiological consequences of such direct and indirect thyroid hormone effects are usually observed at both the heart and arterial levels.

In hyperthyroid patients, increased myocardial contractility, cardiac output and heart rate, shortening of the pre-ejection period, reduction in the pre-ejection period / left ventricular ejection time ratio have been described at the heart level [136-140]. A hyperkinetic arterial circulation consisting of an increase in blood velocity, blood flow, higher peak systolic acceleration, uncommon elevation of diastolic blood pressure and more common systolic hypertension in younger patients and a decrease of total peripheral resistance have been described at the arterial level [141].

In hypothyroid patients, reduction of cardiac output, lengthening of the pre-ejection period (PEP), shortening of the left ventricular ejection time (LVET) and increased PEP/LVET ratios have been observed at the heart level. Elevation of diastolic blood pressure and total peripheral resistance have been described at the arterial level [142].

Considering the above interactions between thyroid hormones and the hemodynamic parameters regulating the PWV principles, it seems evident that any thyroid dysfunction will be expressed by an alteration of the large artery structure or function. Despite this evidence, few, if any, controlled studies have been performed in order to investigate these abnormalities. In fact, at the beginning of this century, Silberman in 1913 [143], using the kymograph, showed very variable PWV values in patients with hyperthyroidism. Sands in 1924 [9] analysed PWV using an optical device on different arteries in a small group ($n = 6$) of patients with hyperthyroidism. He reported a close average but greater variations of PWV values in hyperthyroid groups than in normal individuals, and that PWV with certain limits of cardiovascular disturbance is unchanged in hyperthyroidism. In 1927, Beyerholm [10] analysed carotid-radial PWV in young women with Basedow's disease. The results of this study "seem to indicate that PWV in cases of Basedow's disease keeps within the normal limits as a rule, but on the other hand may be increased without the systolic blood pressure being increased; the pulse frequency does not seem to play any part." More recently, Felt et al. [137] studied PWV in 231 subjects with hyper- and hypothyroidism. Their results showed in younger subjects (20–39 years) that PWV was higher in thyrotoxicosis and lower in hypothyroidism. Changes of PWV in higher age groups were not influenced by increased or reduced thyroid function.

In summary, the interactions between thyroid hormones and cardiovascular hemodynamics suggest an expected change of PWV in patients with thyroid dysfunction. Few studies have been performed in this field; their results suggest, at least in younger patients, that PWV is increased with hyperthyroidism. More specific studies are needed in order to clarify the consequences of thyroid dysfunction in large arteries.

Postmenopausal women

(See also chapter IV, sections on on Age and Gender.)

In the previous chapters, arterial stiffness and PWV have been described to be lower in young women than in young men, whereas similar, if not higher values have been reported in older women by comparison to older men. Moreover, the increase of PWV with age has been described as steeper in women than in men over 45 years old.

London et al. [144] investigated the influence of sex and age in normotensive and hypertensive subjects. Their results showed in premenopausal women lower PWV values at the upper-limb and lower-limb levels than in age-matched men, whereas aortic (carotid-femoral) PWV was not different. In postmenopausal women, PWV values measured at the three different levels did not differ from those in men.

Elsewhere, Maldonado et al. [145] have shown an increase of carotid-femoral PWV in postmenopausal women (natural or surgical menopause) by comparison to age- and blood pressure-matched premenopausal women.

Mori et al. [146] analysed the relationship between aortic PWV and osteoporosis in elderly women. Their results showed significant inverse correlation between PWV and bone mineral content, mainly in the group in which the serum alkaline phosphatase was high.

Recently, we analysed the increase of carotid-femoral PWV with age in hypertensive men and women from the Complior® study (personal data). The results, adjusted for blood pressure level, showed a steeper increase of PWV in women over 55 years old than in men [147].

Athletes

Mellerowicz et al. [148] and Schimmler [149] have analysed aortic PWV in endurance athletes. Their results showed lower PWV values in athletes by comparison to untrained subjects and that the increase of aortic PWV with age was significantly smaller in endurance athletes than in a normal population of untrained adults *(table XII)*. These results may be related to a direct effect of endurance training on the arterial wall or to indirect effects via hemodynamic (blood pressure, heart rate, etc.) or neurohumoral parameters.

TABLE XII. Influence of age and training on aortic PWV. (Adapted from Schimmler [149].)

| Age | Aortic PWV (m/s) | | | |
| | Untrained males | | Endurance athletes | |
	n	mean	*n*	mean
10–19 years	33	6.17	35	6.17
20–29 years	77	6.88	58	6.48*
30–39 years	51	7.41	34	6.71*

n = number, * $p < 0.05$ when compared with values in untrained males.

Vaitkevicius et al. [150] analysed the effect of age and aerobic capacity on arterial stiffness in healthy adults. They showed that PWV varied inversely with VO_2 max, and that arterial compliance and distensibility are increased with physical fitness. Moreover, in endurance trained male athletes, the arterial stiffness indices were significantly reduced relative to their sedentary age peers despite similar blood pressure. Kingwell et al. [151] suggested that these changes might be linked to concomitant alterations in baroreflex sensitivity and that arterial compliance may influence baroreflex function in athletes and hypertensives.

Conversely, Gauthier et al. [152] showed higher PWV measured at the arm in high-level sportsmen by comparison to sedentary subjects; they suggested that this decrease in arterial distensibility might participate in the development of cardiac hypertrophy-dilatation, frequently observed in athletes. More recently, Kool et al. [153] analysed the effects of exercise training on the carotid, brachial and femoral arteries in male cyclists by comparison to sedentary subjects. The vessel wall properties of the carotid artery did not differ between the two groups, whereas the femoral and the brachial arteries were more distensible in the cyclists. In physically active women, Tanaka et al. [154] showed that age-related increases in central arterial stiffness are not observed in highly physically active women and that aerobic fitness is an independent physiological parameter of aortic stiffness.

Hypotension and postural hypotension

Several case reports have been published on PWV and hypotension. Ruschke in 1912 [72] used an optical device to record carotid-radial PWV, Münzer in 1912 [73] used the Kymograph® for the upper arm to calf measurements, Laubry et al. in 1921 [77] used the Kymograph® for the subclavian-radial and femoro-tibial arteries, Ude in 1933 [78] used an optical device to record the subclavian-femoral; all their results showed a decrease in PWV in patients with hypotension by comparison to normal individuals.

In order to test the effect of blood pressure variations on PWV, Haynes et al. in 1936 [11] analysed the carotid-brachial and carotid-radial pulse wave velocities in a few cases of postural hypotension. The arm was kept at heart level and measurements were made with the patients lying and standing. Their results showed a fall in PWV accompanying the fall in blood pressure after standing, whereas the controls showed no significant changes.

More recently, several studies analysed the relationships between PWV, baroreflex sensitivity and autonomic nervous system dysfunction. Thus, Okada et al. in 1992 [155] showed that PWV and heart rate variability may be useful for diagnosing the cardiovascular autonomic neuropathy. In 1995, Siche et al. [156] described a significant correlation between baroreflex sensitivity and carotid-femoral PWV in hypertensive patients which was independent of age and blood pressure levels. Moreover, Okada et al. [28] analysed five indices obtained from PWV recording series performed in healthy subjects and in patients with diabetes or vertigo (the mean and the coefficient of variation during supine rest, those after standing and the change of the mean values before and after standing); their results showed that the change of the mean PWV immediately after standing allows assessment of peripheral vascular sympathetic functions. Elsewhere, Ahlgren et al. [32] showed in women with type 1 diabetes mellitus a significant correlation between increased aortic stiffness (ultrasound technique) and parasympathetic dysfunction (see also chapter IV, section on Heart rate and this chapter, section on Diabetes).

In summary, several studies showed a decrease of PWV in patients with hypotension or postural hypotension. There is increasing evidence that PWV is related to baroreflex sensitivity and that it may be useful for diagnosing some cardiovascular autonomic dysfunction observed in several diseases such as hypertension and diabetes.

Homocysteine

Few studies have reported the influence of homocysteine levels on arterial stiffness. Blacher et al. [123] have shown that carotid-femoral PWV correlated with plasma homocysteine levels, even after adjustments on systolic BP and age in hypertensive subjects. In patients with end-stage renal disease, lower limb PWV was positively and independently correlated with plasma homocysteine levels; no similar correlations were observed at the aortic or the upper-limb levels. Recently, Smilde et al. [157] investigated patients homozygous and heterozygous for cystathionine beta-synthase (CBS) deficiency by comparison to healthy subjects and patients with other cardiovascular risk factors. Their results showed slightly lower values of carotid distensibility in patients homozygous for CBS deficiency; no correlation was found between plasma homocysteine levels and carotid distensibility; plasma homocysteine concentration explained only a small proportion of the distensibility variations of the carotid and to a higher extent of the femoral artery.

Further studies are needed to evaluate the role of homocysteine on arterial stiffness in patients with cardiovascular diseases, and since vitamin supplements are known to decrease plasma homocysteine, their effects on arterial stiffness also need to be evaluated.

REFERENCES

1 Asmar R, Benetos A, London GM, Hughe C, Weiss Y, Topouchian J, et al. Aortic distensibility in normotensive, untreated and treated hypertensive patients. Blood Pressure 1995 ; 4 : 48-54.

2 Eliakim M, Sapoznikov D, Weinman J. PWV in healthy subjects and in patients with various disease states. Am Heart J 1971 ; 82 : 448-57.

3 Safar ME, Girerd X, Laurent S. Structural changes of large conduit arteries in hypertension. Hypertension 1996 ; 14 : 545-55.

4 McDonald DA. Blood flow in arteries: theorical, experimental and clinical principles, 4th ed. London: Arnold; 1998. p. 77-142, 216-69, 283-359, 398-437.

5 Girerd X, Chanudet X, Larroque P, Clement R, Laloux B, Safar ME. Early arterial modifications in young patients with borderline hypertension. J Hypertens 1989 ; 7 Suppl 1 : 456-7.

6 Glen SK, Elliott HL, Curzio JL, Lees KR, Reid JL. White-coat hypertension as a cause of cardiovascular dysfunction. Lancet 1996 ; 348 : 654-7.

7 Soma J, Aakhus S, Dahl K, Slørdahl S, Wiseth R, Widerøe TE, et al. Hemodynamics in white coat hypertension compared to ambulatory hypertension and normotension. Am J Hypertens 1996 ; 9 : 1090-8.

8 Lantelme P, Milon H, Gharib C, Gayet C, Fortrat JO. White coat effect and reactivity to stress. Cardiovascular and autonomic nervous system responses. Hypertension 1998 ; 31 : 1021-9.

9 Sands J. Studies in pulse wave velocity. III. Pulse wave velocity in pathological conditions. Am J Physiol 1924 ; 71 : 519.

10 Beyerholm O. Studies of the velocity of transmission of the pulse wave velocity in different pathological conditions (principally arteriosclerosis with and without hypertonia, and heart arrhythmiae). Acta Med Scand 1927 ; 67 : 323.

11 Haynes FW, Ellis LB, Weiss S. Pulse wave velocity and arterial elasticity in arterial hypertension, arteriosclerosis and related conditions. Am Heart J 1936 ; 11 : 385-401.

12 Avolio AP. Pulse wave velocity and hypertension. In: Safar ME, ed., Arterial and venous systems in essential hypertension. Martinus Nijhoff ; 1987, p. 133-52.

13 Gribbin B, Pickering TG, Sleight P. Arterial distensibility in normal and hypertensive man. Clin Sci 1979 ; 56 : 413-7.

14 Girerd X, Mourad JJ, Copie X, Moulin C, Acar C, Safar ME, et al. Noninvasive detection of an increased vascular mass in untreated hypertensive patients. Am J Hypertens 1994 ; 7 : 1076-84.

15 Laurent S. Arterial wall hypertrophy and stiffness in essential hypertensive patients. Hypertension 1995 ; 26 : 355-62.

16 Smulyan H, Vardan S, Griffiths A, Gribbin B. Forearm arterial distensibility in systolic hypertension. J Am Coll Cardiol 1984 ; 3 : 3387-93.

17 Pannier BM, Cambillau MS, Vellaud V, Atger V, Moatti N, Safar ME. Abnormalities of lipid metabolism and arterial rigidity in young subjects with borderline hypertension. Clin Invest Med 1993 ; 17 : 42-51.

18 Simon AC, Levenson J, Bouthier J, Safar ME, Avolio AP. Evidence of early degenerative changes in large arteries in human essential hypertension. Hypertension 1985 ; 7 : 675-80.

19 Armentano R, Simon A, Levenson J, Chau NP, Megnien JL, Pichel R. Mechanical pressure versus intrinsic effects of hypertension on large arteries in humans. Hypertension 1991 ; 18 : 657-64.

20 Asmar R, Benetos A, Topouchian J, Laurent P, Panier B, Brisac, et al. Assessment of arterial distensibility by automatic pulse wave velocity measurement. Validation and clinical application studies. Hypertension 1995 ; 26 : 485-90.

21 Lax H, Feinberg AW. Abnormalities of the arterial pulse wave in young diabetic subjects. Circulation 1959 ; 20 : 1106.

22 Woolam GL, Schnur PL, Vallbona C, Hoff HE. The pulse wave velocity as an early indicator of atherosclerosis in diabetic subjects. Circulation 1962 ; 25 : 533-9.

23 Stella A, Gessaroli M, Cifiello BI, Salardi S, Reggiani A, Cacciari E, et al. Elastic modulus in young diabetic patients (ultrasound measurements of PWV). Angiology 1984 ; 35 : 729-34.

24 Christensen T, Neubauer B. Arterial wall stiffness in insulin-dependent diabetes mellitus. An in-vivo study. Acta Radiol 1987 ; 28 : 207-8.

25 Paillole C, Dahan M, Jaeger P, Passa P, Gourgon R. Physical properties of the aorta in normotensive insulin-dependent diabetic subjects. Study using Doppler echocardiography. Arch Mal Cœur Vaiss 1989 ; 82 : 1185-9.

26 Oxlund H, Rasmussen LM, Andreassen TT, Heickendorff L. Increased aortic stiffness in patients with type 1 (insulin-dependent) diabetes mellitus. Diabetologia 1989 ; 32 : 748-52.

27 Krause M, Ederer G, Regling B, Holker S, Bartels H. Early detection of changes in peripheral blood vessels in children and adolescents with insulin-dependent diabetes mellitus using Doppler ultrasound. Monatsschr Kinderheilkd 1991 ; 139 : 282-6.

28 Okada M, Matsuto T, Satoh S, Igarashi S, Baba M, Sugita O, et al. Role of pulse wave velocity for assessing autonomic nervous system activities in reference to heart rate variability. Med Inform (Lond) 1996 ; 21 Suppl 1 : 81-90.

29 Lehmann ED, Gosling RG, Sönksen PH. Arterial wall compliance in diabetes. Diabet Med 1992 ; 9 : 114-9.

30 Kool MJ, Lambert J, Stehouwer CD, Hoeks AP, Struijker Boudier HA, Van Bortel LM. Vessel wall properties of large arteries in uncomplicated IDDM. Diabetes Care 1995 ; 18 : 618-24.

31 Ryden-Ahlgren A, Lane T, Wollmer P, Sonesson B, Hansen F, Sundkvist G. Increased arterial stiffness in women, but not in men, with IDDM. Diabetologia 1995 ; 38 : 1082-9.

32 Ryden-Ahlgren A, Sundkvist G, Wollmer P, Sonesson B, Lanne T. Increased aortic stiffness in

women with type 1 diabetes mellitus is associated with diabetes duration and autonomic nerve function. Diabet Med 1999 ; 16 Suppl 4 : 291-7.

33 Lambert J, Smulders RA, Aarsen M, Gallay FP, Stehouver CD. The acute effect of hyperglycaemia on vessel wall properties. Scand J Clin Lab Invest 1997 ; 57 : 409-14.

34 Jensen-Urstad K, Reichard P, Jensen-Urstad M. Decreased heart rate variability in patients with type 1 diabetes mellitus is related to arterial wall stiffness. J Intern Med 1999 ; 245 : 57-61.

35 Scarpello JH, Martin TR, Ward JD. Ultrasound measurements of pulse-wave velocity in the peripheral arteries of diabetic subjects. Clin Sci 1980 ; 58 : 53-7.

36 Relf IR, Lo CS, Myers KA, Wahlqvist ML. Risk factors for changes in aorto-iliac arterial compliance in healthy men. Arteriosclerosis 1986 ; 6 : 105-8.

37 Lo CS, Relf IR, Myers KA, Wahlqvist ML. Doppler ultrasound recognition of preclinical changes in arterial wall in diabetic subjects: compliance and pulse-wave damping. Diabetes Care 1986 ; 9 : 27-31.

38 Wahlqvist ML, Relf IR, Myers KA, Lo Cs. Diabetes and macrovascular disease: risk factors for atherogenesis and non-invasive investigation of arterial disease. Hum Nutr Clin Nutr 1984 ; 38 : 175-84.

39 Wahlqvist ML, Lo CS, Myers KA, Simpson RW, Simpson JM. Putative determinants of arterial wall compliance in NIDDM. Diabetes Care 1988 ; 11 : 787-90.

40 Megnien JL, Simon A, Valensi P, Flaud P, Merli I, Levenson J. Comparative effects of diabetes mellitus and hypertension on physical properties of human large arteries. J Am Coll Cardiol 1992 ; 20 : 1562-8.

41 Amar J, Chamontin B, Pelissier M, Garelli I, Salvador M. Influence of glucose metabolism on nycthemeral blood pressure variability in hypertensives with an elevated waist-hip ratio. A link with arterial distensibility. Am J Hypertens 1995 ; 8 : 426-8.

42 Tanokuchi S, Okada S, Ota Z. Factors related to aortic pulse-wave velocity in patients with non-insulin-dependent diabetes mellitus. J Int Med Res 1995 ; 23 : 423-30.

43 Hopkins KD, Lehmann ED, Jones RL, Turay RC, Gosling RG. A family history of NIDDM is associated with decreased aortic distensibility in normal healthy young adult subjects. Diabetes Care 1996 ; 19 : 501-3.

44 Emoto M, Nishizawa Y, Kawagishi T, Maekawa K, Hiura Y, Kanda H, et al. Stiffness indices beta of the common carotid and femoral arteries are associated with insulin resistance in NIDDM. Diabetes Care 1998 ; 21 : 1178-82.

45 Gosling RG, Hayes JA, Segre-Mackay W. Induction of atheroma in cockerels as a model for studying alterations in blood flow. J Atheroscler Res 1969 ; 9 : 47-56.

46 Newman DL, Gosling RG, Bowden NLR. Changes in aortic distensibility and area ratio with the development of atherosclerosis. Atherosclerosis 1971 ; 14 : 231-40.

47 Farrar DJ, Green HP, Bond MG, Wagner WP, Gobbee RA. Aortic pulse wave velocity, elasticity and composition in a non-human primate model of atherosclerosis. Circ Res 1978 ; 43 : 52-62.

48 Manning PJ, Clarkson TB. Development, distribution, and lipid content of diet-induced atherosclerotic lesions of rhesus monkeys. Exp Mol Pathol 1972 ; 17 : 38-54.

49 Hirai T, Sasayama S, Kawasaki T, Yagi S. Stiffness of systemic arteries in patients with myocardial infarction. Circulation 1989 ; 80 : 78-86.

50 Jenkins PJ, Harper RW, Nestel PJ. Severity of coronary atherosclerosis related to lipoprotein concentration. Br Med J 1978 ; 2 : 388-91.

51 Blacher J, Asmar R, Djane S, London GM, Safar ME. Aortic pulse wave velocity as a marker of cardiovascular risk in hypertensive patients. Hypertension 1999 ; 33 : 1111-7.

52 Avolio AP, Fa-Quan D, Wei-Qiang L, Yao-Fei L, Zhen-Dong H, Lian-Fen X, et al. Effects of aging on arterial distensibility in populations with high and low prevalence of hypertension: comparison between urban and rural communities in China. Circulation 1985 ; 71 : 202-10.

53 Schimmler W. Untersuchungen zu elastizitatsproblemen der Aorta. Arch Kreislaufforschung 1965 ; 47 : 189-233.

54 Avolio A, O'Rourke M, Clyde K, Simmons L. Change of arterial distensibility with age in subjects with familial hypercholesterolemia. Aust NZ J Med 1985 ; Suppl II : 56.

55 Lehmann ED, Watts GF, Fatemi-Langroudi B, Gosling RG. Aortic compliance in young patients with heterozygous familial hypercholesterolaemia. Clin Sci 1992 ; 83 : 717-21.

56 Blankenhorm DH, Krausch DM. Reversal of atherosis and sclerosis; the two components of atherosclerosis. Circulation 1989 ; 79 : 1-7.

57 Lehmann E, Watts G, Gosling R. Aortic distensibility and hypercholesterolaemia. Lancet 1992 ; 340 : 1171-2.

58 Lehmann E, Hopkins K, Parker J, Gosling R. Hyperlipidaemia, hypertension and coronary heart disease. Lancet 1995 ; 345 : 862-3.

59 Relf IRN, Lo CS, Myers KA, Wahlqvist ML. Risk factors for changes in aorto-iliac arterial compliance in healthy men. Arteriosclerosis 1986 ; 6 :105-8.

60 London GM, Guerin AP, Marchais SJ, Pannier B, Safar ME, Day M, et al. Cardiac and arterial interactions in end-stage renal disease. Kidney Int 1996 ; 50 : 600-8.

61 London GM, Marchais SJ, Safar ME, Genest AF, Guerin AP, Metivier F, et al. Aortic and large artery compliance in end-stage renal failure. Kidney Int 1990 ; 37 : 137-42.

62 Dart AM, Lacombe F, Yeoh JK, Cameron JD, Jennings GL, Laufer E, et al. Aortic distensibility in patients with isolated hypercholesterolemia, coronary artery disease, or cardiac transplant. Lancet 1991 ; 338 : 270-3.

63 Barenbrock M, Spieker C, Kerber S, Vielhauer C, Hoeks APG, Zidek W, et al. Different effects of hypertension, atherosclerosis and hyperlipidaemia on arterial distensibility. J Hypertens 1995 ; 13 : 1712-7.

64 Cameron JD, Jennings GL, Dart AM. The relationship between arterial compliance, age, blood pressure and serum lipid levels. J Hypertens 1995 ; 13 : 1718-23.

65 Kupari M, Hekali P, Keto P, Poutanen VP, Tikkanen MJ, Standerstkjold-Nordenstam CG, et al. Relation of aortic stiffness to factors modifying the risk of atherosclerosis in healthy people. Arterioscler Thromb 1994 ; 14 : 386-94.

66 Moritani T, Crouse SF, Shea CH, Davidson N, Nakamura E. Arterial pulse wave velocity, Fourier pulsatility index, and blood lipid profiles. Med Sci Sports Exerc 1987 ; 19 : 404-9.

67 Giral P, Atger V, Amar J, Cambillau M, Del Pino M, Megnien JL, et al. A relationship between aortic stiffness and serum HDL3 cholesterol concentrations in hypercholesterolaemic, symptom-free men. The PCVMETRA Group (Groupe de Prévention Cardiovasculaire en Médecine du Travail). J Cardiovasc Risk 1994 ; 1 : 53-8.

68 Pitsavos C, Toutouzas K, Dernellis J, Skoumas J, Skoumbourdis E, Stefanadis C, et al. Aortic stiffness in young patients with heterozygous familial hypercholesterolemia. Am Heart J 1998 ; 135 : 604-8.

69 Iannuzzi A, Rubba P, Pauciullo P, Celentano E, Capano G, Sartorio R, et al. Stiffness of the aortic wall in hypercholesterolemic children. Metabolism 1999 ; 48 : 55-9.

70 Friberger R. Ueber die Pulswellengeschwindigkeit bei Arterien mit fülhlbarer Wandverdickung. Dtsch Arch Klin Med 1912 ; 107 : 280.

71 Eismayer G, Saeger W. Die Pulswellengeschiwindigkeit in verschiedenen Gefässgebieten; die Pulswellengeschwindigkeit in verschiedenen Gefässgebieten bei Kreislaufgesunden im Ruhezustand und unter Einwirkung von Medikamenten. Z Ges Exper Med 1934 ; 96 : 233.

72 Turner RH, Herrmann GR. Pulse wave velocity under varying conditions in normal and abnormal human cardiovascular systems. J Clin Invest 1927 ; 4 : 430.

73 Ruschke. Beitrag z. Lehre von des Fortpflanzungsgeschwindigkeit der Pulsewellen bei gesunden und kranken Individuen [dissertation]. Jena ; 1912.

74 Münzer E. Die Fortpflanzungsgeschwindigkeit der Pulswellen in gesunden und krankhaftveränderten Blutgefässen. Verh Dtsch Kong Inn Med 1912 ; 29 : 431.

75 Bazett HC, Dreyer NB. Measurements of pulse wave velocity. Am J Physiol, 1922 ; 63 : 94-109.

76 Bramwell JC, Hill AV. Velocity of transmission of the pulse wave and elasticity of arteries. Lancet 1922 ; 1 : 891.

77 Silberman. Ueber Pulswellengeschwindigkeit und ihre diagnostische Bedeutung. Zentralbl Herz Gefässkrank 1913 ; 5 : 297.

78 Laubry C, Mougeot A, Giroux R. La vitesse de propagation de l'onde pulsatile artérielle. Arch Mal Cœur Vaiss 1921 ; 14 : 49.

79 Ude H. Die Beurteilung der Windkesselfunktion des Aorta mit Hilfe der Pulswellengeschwindigkeit. Klinik Wehnsehr 1933 ; 12 : 1484.

80 Lehmann ED, Gosling RG, Parker JR, de Silva T, Taylor MG. A blood pressure independent index of aortic distensibility. Br J Radiol 1993 ; 66 : 126-31.

81 Nishio S, Harima M, Kobayagawa H. Clinical study of risk factors concerning arteriosclerosis of the patients undergoing hemodialysis. Hinyokika Kiyo 1990 ; 36 : 645-8.

82 Asai K, Miura S, Kawahara H, Toriyama T, Kuzuya F. A comparative study of atherosclerosis and osteopenia in elderly and young hemodialysis patients. Aging (Milano) 1991 ; 3 : 79-87.

83 Taniwaki H, Nishizawa Y, Kawagishi T, Ishimura E, Emoto, M Okamura T, et al. Decrease in glomerular filtration rate in Japanese patients with type 2 diabetes is linked to atherosclerosis. Diabetes Care 1998 ; 21 : 1848-55.

84 Blacher J, Djane S, Asmar R, Safar M. Déterminants de la rigidité artérielle chez le sujet âgé. Arch Mal Cœur 1997 ; 90 : 35.

85 Dart AM, Qi XL. Determinants of arterial stiffness in Chinese migrants to Australia. Atherosclerosis 1995 ; 117 : 263-72.

86 Namekata T, Moore D, Suzuki K, Mori M, Hatano S, Hayashi C, et al. A study of the association between the aortic pulse wave velocity and atherosclerotic risk factors among Japanese Americans in Seattle, USA. Nippon Koshu Eisei Zasshi 1997 ; 44 : 942-51.

87 Akisaka M, Ashitomi I, Adachi M, Tanaka Y, Suzuki M. The relationship between aortic pulse wave velocity and atherogenic index in centenarians. Nippon Ronen Igakkai Zasshi 1993 ; 30 : 467-73.

88 Van Popele N, Grobbee DE, Bots ML, Asmar R, Topouchian J, Hofman A, et al. Association between atherosclerosis and arterial stiffness in an elderly population. In: 17th Scientific Meeting of the International Society of Hypertension. Workshop on Arterial Structure and Function, Amsterdam: 1998.

89 Simonson E, Nakagawa K. Effect of age on pulse wave velocity and "aortic ejection time" in healthy men and in men with coronary artery disease. Circulation 1960 ; 22 : 126-9.

90 Hirai T, Sasayama S, Kawasaki T, Yagi SI. Stiffness of systemic arteries in patients with myocardial infarction. A noninvasive method to predict severity of coronary atherosclerosis. Circulation 1989 ; 80 : 78-86.

91 Bogren HG, Mohiaddin RH, Klipstein RK, Firmin DN, Underwood RS, Rees SR, et al. The function of the aorta in ischemic heart disease: a magnetic resonance and angiographic study of aortic compliance and blood flow patterns. Am Heart J 1989 ; 118 : 234-47.

92 Ouchi Y, Terashita K, Nakamura T, Yamaoki K, Yazaki Y, Toda E, et al. Aortic pulse wave velocity

in patients with coronary atherosclerosis – a comparison with coronary angiographic findings. Nippon Ronen Igakkai Zasshi 1991 ; 28 : 40-5.

93 Airaksinen KE, Salmela PI, Linnaluoto MK, Ikaheimo MJ, Ahola K, Ryhanen LJ. Diminished arterial elasticity in diabetes: association with fluorescent advanced glycosylation end products in collagen. Cardiovasc Res 1993 ; 27 : 942-5.

94 Triposkiadis F, Kallikazaros I, Trikas A, Stefanadis C, Stratos C, Tsekoura D, et al. A comparative study of the effect of coronary artery disease on ascending and abdominal aorta distensibility and PWV. Acta Cardiol 1993 ; 48 : 221-33.

95 Megnien JL, Simon A, Denarie N, Del-Pino M, Gariepy J, Segond P, et al. Aortic stiffening does not predict coronary and extracoronary atherosclerosis in asymptomatic men at risk for cardiovascular disease. Am J Hypertens 1998 ; 11 : 293-301.

96 Gatzka CD, Cameron JD, Kingwell BA, Dart AM. Relation between coronary artery disease, aortic stiffness, and left ventricular structure in a population sample. Hypertension 1998 ; 32 : 575-8.

97 Neil-Dwyer G, Bartlett JR, Nicholls AC, Narcisi P, Pope FM. Collagen deficiency and ruptured cerebral aneurysms. A clinical and biochemical study. J Neurosurg 1983 ; 59 : 16-20.

98 Neil-Dwyer G, Child AH, Dorrance DE, Pope FM, Bartlett J. Aortic compliance in patients with ruptured intracranial aneurysms. Lancet 1983 ; 23 : 939-40.

99 Adamson J, Humphries SE, Ostergaard JR, Voldby B, Richards P, Powell JT. Are cerebral aneurysms atherosclerotic? Stroke 1994 ; 25 : 963-6.

100 Ostergaard JR, Oxlund H. Collagen type III deficiency in patients with rupture of intracranial vascular aneurysms. J Neurosurg 1987 ; 67 : 690-6.

101 Lehmann ED, Hopkins KD, Jones RL, Rudd Ag, Gosling RG. Aortic distensibility in patients with cerebrovascular disease. Clin Sci 1995 ; 89 : 247-53.

102 Arnold JM, Marchiori GE, Imrie JR, Burton GL, Pflugfelder PW, Kostuk WJ. Large artery function in patients with chronic heart failure. Circulation 1991 ; 84 ; 2418-25.

103 Lage SG, Kopel L, Monachini MC, Medeiros CJ, Pileggi F, Polak JF, et al. Carotid arterial compliance in patients with congestive heart failure secondary to idiopathic dilated cardiomyopathy. Am J Cardiol 1994 ; 74 : 691-5.

104 Ramsey MW, Goodfellow J, Jones CJ, Luddington LA, Lewis MJ, Henderson AH. Endothelial control of arterial distensibility is impaired in chronic heart failure. Circulation 1995 ; 92 : 3212-9.

105 Giannattasio C, Failla M, Stella ML, Mangoni AA, Carugo S, Pozzi M, et al. Alterations of radial artery compliance in patients with congestive heart failure. Am J Cardiol 1995 ; 76 : 381-5.

106 Potocka-Plazak K, Kolasa R, Poplawski T, Kulczycka J, Plazak W. Correlation between aortic pulse wave velocity and norepinephrine, epinephrine, aldosterone and plasma renin activity in very elderly patients and in patients with congestive heart failure. Aging (Milano) 1998 ; 1 : 48-52.

107 Safar ME, Laurent S, Asmar RG, Safavian A, London GM. Systolic hypertension in patients with arteriosclerosis obliterans of the lower limbs. Angiology 1987 ; 38 : 287-95.

108 Simonson E, Koff S, Keys A, Minckler J. Contour of the toe pulse, reactive hyperemia, and pulse transmission velocity: group and repeat variability, effect of age, exercise, and disease. Am Heart J 1955 ; 50 : 260-79.

109 Hirata K, Triposkiadis F, Sparks E, Bowen J, Wooley CF, Boudoulas H. The Marfan syndrome: abnormal aortic elastic properties. J Am Coll Cardiol 1991 ; 18 : 57-63.

110 Jeremy RW, Huang H, Hwa J, McCarron H, Hughes CF, Richards JG. Relation between age, arterial distensibility, and aortic dilatation in the Marfan syndrome. Am J Cardiol 1994 ; 74 : 369-73.

111 Groenink M, de Roos A, Mulder BJ, Spaan JA, Van der Wall EE. Changes in aortic distensibility and pulse wave velocity assessed with magnetic resonance imaging following beta-blocker therapy in the Marfan syndrome. Am J Cardiol 1998 ; 82 : 203-8.

112 Jondeau G, Boutouyrie P, Lacolley P, Laloux B, Dubourg O, Bourdarias JP. Central pulse pressure is a major determinant of ascending aorta dilation in Marfan's syndrome. Circulation 1999 ; 99 : 2677-81.

113 Yin FCP, Brin KP, Ting CT, Pyeritz RE. Arterial hemodynamic indices in Marfan's syndrome. Circulation 1989 ; 79 : 854-62.

114 Matton MT, De Paepe A, De Keyser F, François B. Unusual familial manifestation of Ehlers-Danlos syndrome. Prog Clin Biol Res 1982 ; 104 : 243-58.

115 François B, De Paepe A, Matton MT, Clement D. pulse wave velocity recordings in a family with ecchymotic Ehlers-Danlos syndrome. Int Angiol 1986 ; 5 : 1-5.

116 Sonesson B, Hansen F, Lanne T. The mechanical properties of elastic arteries in Ehlers-Danlos syndrome. Eur J Vasc Endovasc Surg 1997 ; 14 : 258-64.

117 MacSweeney ST, Young G, Greenhalgh RM, Powell JT. Mechanical properties of the aneurysmal aorta. Br J Surg 1992 ; 79 : 1281-4.

118 Vorp DA, Mandarino WA, Webster MW, Gorcsan J 3rd. Potential influence of intraluminal thrombus on abdominal aortic aneurysm as assessed by a new non-invasive method. Cardiovasc Surg 1996 ; 4 : 732-9.

119 Boutouyrie P, Glaser C, Moryusef A, Bézie Y, Fabiani JN, Laurent S, et al. Viscoelastic properties of large arteries and extracellular matrix composition in patients with abdominal aortic aneurysm. Thérapie 1999 ; 54 : 85-91.

120 London G, Guerin A, Pannier B, Marchais S, Benetos A, Safar M. Increased systolic pressure in chronic uremia. Role of arterial wave reflections. Hypertension 1992 ; 20 : 10-9.

121 Amar J, Chamontin B, Vernier I, Lenfant V, Conte J, Salvador M. Arterial blood pressure changes, circadian rhythm and arterial elasticity in hemo-

dialysed patients. Arch Mal Cœur Vaiss 1994 ; 87 : 921-4.

122 Demuth K, Blacher J, Guerin AP, Benoit MO, Moatti N, Safar ME. Endothelin and cardiovascular remodelling in end-stage renal disease. Nephrol Dial Transplant 1998 ; 13 : 375-83.

123 Blacher J, Demuth K, Guerin AP, Safar ME, Moatti N, London G. Influence of biochemical alterations on arterial stiffness in patients with end-stage renal disease. Arterioscler Thromb Vasc Biol 1998 ; 18 : 535-41.

124 Shoji T, Nishizawa Y, Kawagishi T, Kawazaki K, Taniwaki H, Tabata T, et al. Intermediate-density lipoprotein as an independent risk factor for aortic atherosclerosis in hemodialysis patients. J Am Soc Nephrol 1998 ; 9 : 1277-84.

125 Kishimoto T, Terada T, Yamagami S, Sugimura T, Nishio S, Maekawa M. Correlation between blood prostaglandins, plasma lipids and atherosclerosis in dialyzed patients. Blood Purif 1990 ; 8 : 141-8.

126 Blacher J, Pannier B, Guerin AP, Marchais SJ, Safar ME, London GM. Carotid arterial stiffness as a predictor of cardiovascular and all-cause mortality in end-stage renal disease. Hypertension 1998 ; 32 : 570-4.

127 Markussis V, Beshyah SA, Fisher C, Sharp P, Nicolaides AN, Johnston DG. Detection of premature atherosclerosis by high-resolution ultrasonography in symptom-free hypopituitary adults. Lancet 1992 ; 340 : 1188-92.

128 Markussis V, Beshyah SA, Fisher C, Parker KH, Nicolaides AN, Johnston DG. Abnormal carotid arterial wall dynamics in symptom-free hypopituitary adults. Eur J Endocrinol 1997 ; 136 : 157-64.

129 Lehmann ED, Hopkins KD, Weissberger AJ, Gosling RC, Sönksen PH. Aortic distensibility in growth hormone deficiency. Lancet 1993 ; 341 : 309.

130 Pfeifer M, Verhovec R, Zizek B, Prezelj J, Poredos P, Clayton RN. Growth hormone (GH) treatment reverses early atherosclerotic changes in GH-deficient adults. J Clin Endocrinol Metab 1999 ; 84 : 453-7.

131 Brunel P, Girerd X, Laurent S, Pannier B, Safar M. Acute changes in forearm haemodynamics produced by cigarette smoking in healthy normotensive non-smokers are not influenced by propanolol or pindolol. Eur J Clin Pharmacol 1992 ; 42 Suppl 2 : 143-6.

132 Berlin I, Cournot A, Renout P, Duchier J, Safar M. Peripheral haemodynamic effects of smoking in habitual smokers. A methodological study. Eur J Clin Pharmacol 1990 ; 38 Suppl 1 : 57-60.

133 Failla M, Grappiolo A, Carugo S, Calchera I, Giannattasio C, Mancia G. Effects of cigarette smoking on carotid and radial artery distensibility. J Hypertens 1997 ; 15 Suppl 12 : 1659-64.

134 Levenson J, Simon AC, Cambien FA, Beretti C. Cigarette smoking and hypertension. Factors independently associated with blood hyperviscosity and arterial rigidity. Arteriosclerosis 1987 ; 7 Suppl 6 : 572-7.

135 Nakamoto A, Kawanishi M, Hiraoka M, Matsuoka S, Konemori G, Itoh M, et al. The effect of smoking on aortic pulse wave velocity using a new method for data analysis. Nippon Ronen Igakkai Zasshi 1989 ; 26 Suppl 1 : 26-30.

136 Polikar R, Burger AG, Scherrer U, Nicod P. The thyroid and the heart. Circulation 1993 ; 87 Suppl 5 : 1435-41.

137 Felt V, Cenkova V. Thyroid hormones and arterial distensibility in man. Czech Med 1984 ; 7 Suppl 2 : 90-9.

138 Saito I, Saruta T. Hypertension in thyroid disorders. Endocrinol Metab Clin North Am 1994 ; 23 Suppl 2 : 379-86.

139 Senda Y, Nishibu M, Kawai K, Mizukami Y, Hashimoto T. Evaluation of type IV collagen in patients with various thyroid disease. Rinsho Byori 1993 ; 41 Suppl 12 : 1338-42.

140 Galloe AM, Rolff M, Nordin H, Ladefoged SD, Mogensen NB. Cardiac performance and thyroid function. The correlation between systolic time intervals, heart rate and thyroid hormone levels. Dan Med Bull 1993 ; 40 Suppl 4 : 492-5.

141 Chemla D, Levenson J, Valensi P, Lecarpentier Y, Pourny JC, Pithois-Merli I, et al. Effect of beta adrenoceptors and thyroid hormones on velocity and acceleration of peripheral arterial flow in hyperthyroidism. Am J Cardiol 1990 ; 65 Suppl 7 : 494-500.

142 Saito I, Ito K, Swuita T. Hypothyroidism as a cause of hypertension. Hypertension 1983 ; 5 : 112-5.

143 Silberman. Ueber Pulswellengeschwindigkeit und ihre Diagnostische Bedeutung. Zentralbl Herz Gefässkrank 1913 ; 5 : 297.

144 London J, Marchais AP, Marchais SJ, Pannier B, Safar ME, Stimpel M. Influence of sex on arterial hemodynamics and blood pressure. Role of body height. Hypertension 1995 ; 26 : 514-9.

145 Maldonado J, Aguas Lopes F, Barbosa A, Alves Z, Pego M, Texeira F, et al. Circadian blood pressure profile, variability and arterial distensibility in postmenopausal women before and after hormonal replacement therapy. Am J Hypertens 1998 ; 11 : 95A.

146 Mori H, Seto S, Oku Y, Hashiba K, Ochi S, Seto M, et al. The relationship between the aortic PWV and osteoporosis in elderly women. Nippon Ronen Igakkai Zasshi 1991 ; 28 : 200-4.

147 Asmar R, Topouchian J, Pannier B, Rudnichi A, Safar M. Reversion of arterial abnormalities by long-term antihypertensive therapy in a large population. The Complior® study. J Hypertens 1999 ; 17 Suppl 3 : S9.

148 Mellerowicz, Peterman. Z Kreisl-Forsch 1956 ; 45 : 716.

149 Schimmler, Wegner. Z Kreisl-Forsch 1972 ; 61 : 648.

150 Vaitkevicius PB, Fleg JL, Engel JH, O'Connor F, Wright JG, Lakatta LE, et al. Effects of age and aerobic capacity on arterial stiffness in healthy adults. Circulation 1993 ; 88 : 1456-62.

151 Kingwell BA, Cameron JD, Gillies KJ, Jennings GL, Dart AM. Arterial compliance may influence

baroreflex function in athletes and hypertensives. Am J Physiol 1995 ; 268 : 411-8.

152 Gauthier PJ, Chibatte F. Value of the measurement of pulse wave velocity in high level sportsmen. Practical applications. Arch Mal Cœur Vaiss 1989 ; 2 : 29-33.

153 Kool MJ, Struijker-Boudier HA, Wijnen JA, Hoeks AP, Van Bortel LM. Effects of diurnal variability and exercise training on properties of large arteries. J Hypertens 1992 ; 10 Suppl : 49-52.

154 Tanaka H, DeSouza CA, Seals DR. Absence of age-related increase in central arterial stiffness in physically active women. Arterioscler Thromb Vasc Biol 1998 ; 18 : 127-32.

155 Okada M, Matsuto T, Sugita O, Yamada T. Use of heart rate variability and pulse wave velocity for diagnosing cardiovascular autonomic neuropathy. Rinsho Byori 1992 ; 40 Suppl 6 : 655-9.

156 Siche JP, Chevallier M, Tremel F, de Gaudemaris R, Boutelant S, Comparat V, et al. Baroreflex sensitivity and vascular involvement in hyper- tension. Arch Mal Cœur Vaiss 1995 ; 88 Suppl 8 : 1243-6.

157 Smilde TJ, van den Berkmortel FW, Boers GH, Wollersheim H, de Boo T, van Langen H, et al. Carotid and femoral artery wall thickness and stiffness in patients at risk for cardiovascular disease, with special emphasis on hyperhomocysteinemia. Arterioscler Thromb Vasc Biol 1998 ; 18 : 1958-63.

CHAPTER

Pulse wave velocity and prognosis

In order to evaluate the prognostic value of PWV and arterial stiffness, different approaches need to be analysed. These approaches must look at various aspects, ranging from the determinants of PWV to its value as independent predictor of morbidity and mortality.

CARDIOVASCULAR RISK FACTORS

(See also chapter IV on Factors influencing PWV.)

Several studies performed in various populations showed significant correlations or powerful interactions between PWV and the so called 'major' cardiovascular risk factors, such as age, gender, hypertension, diabetes, and smoking.

Significant interactions between PWV and the so-called 'minor' cardiovascular risk factors have also been established, as with pulse pressure, heart rate, waist circumference and waist/hip ratio, left ventricular hypertrophy, microalbuminuria, homocysteine, and sedentariness.

Most of these associations between PWV and the major and minor cardiovascular risk factors have been described either independently or persist after adjustment on the other factors (see previous chapters).

ORGAN DAMAGE – SURROGATE MARKERS

Pulse wave velocity and microalbuminuria

Despite some reports on the association between renal function and PWV, few studies have analysed the relationships between PWV and microalbuminuria. Takegoshi et al. [1] found faster PWV in diabetics with microalbuminuria than those without, and showed significant correlation between PWV and urinary albumin. They concluded that PWV may be a reliable index of diabetic micro- and macroangiopathy as expressed by microalbuminuria. Elsewhere, Taniwaki et al. [2] investigated patients with type 2 diabetes and found arterial stiffness to be an independent factor associated with the glomerular filtration rate.

Pulse wave velocity and arterial atherosclerosis

Several studies have highlighted the associations between PWV and different arterial atherosclerosis surrogate markers, such as aortic calcification index, carotid intima-medial thickness and ankle/brachial systolic pressure index.

PWV has been found to be increased in different populations with various arterial diseases, such as in patients with coronary heart disease, cerebrovascular disease or with lower limb obliterans atherosclerosis.

Pulse wave velocity and left ventricular hypertrophy

It is well established that the development and regression of cardiac hypertrophy in hypertension do not depend exclusively on the level of blood pressure, but are also modulated by various neurohumoral factors and the aortic properties. Indeed, the elevation in blood pressure is usually considered to reflect the elevation in total peripheral resistance; however, this increase in afterload may also be related to the reduction in arterial distensibility.

In fact, reduced arterial distensibility has been shown to be responsible for a disproportionate increase in systolic BP, which is an important component of left ventricular stress.

In this regard, Bouthier et al. [3] analysed in normotensive and hypertensive subjects the relationship between carotid-femoral PWV and echocardiographic parameters such as left ventricular mass-volume ratio and left ventricular end-systolic stress. Their results showed highly significant correlations between carotid-femoral PWV and the left ventricular mass-volume ratio, and between PWV and end-systolic stress, even after adjustment for age (figure 1). These results suggested that aortic distensibility, assessed by carotid-femoral PWV, plays an important role in the left ventricular load, hypertrophy and hemodynamic.

More recently, several authors highlighted the interactions between aortic distensibility, carotid intima-medial thickness and left ventricular structure and function in various populations [4-6].

PULSE WAVE VELOCITY AS A MARKER

Several prospective longitudinal studies to evaluate PWV as a marker of morbidity and mortality are in process. Nevertheless, a certain amount of data in this field are available and allow some considerations to be drawn in different prognotic approaches.

Pulse wave velocity as a marker of atherosclerosis

Several studies have shown close correlations between PWV and atherosclerosis. Increased PWV has been found in populations with various arterial alterations. Recently, Van Popele et al. [7] showed close correlations between carotid-femoral PWV

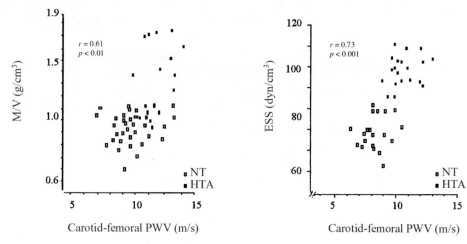

FIGURE 1. Correlations between carotid-femoral pulse wave velocity, left ventricular mass/volume ratio (M/V) and left ventricular end-systolic stress (ESS) in normotensive (NT) and hypertensive (HT) subjects. (Adapted from Bouthier et al. [3].)

and other indicators of atherosclerosis in the elderly population of the Rotterdam study. Lehmann et al. [8, 9] investigated patients with vascular disease and/or diabetes mellitus. Their results revealed that patients with the greatest number of cardiovascular risk factors and events had the stiffest aortas (calculated on the basis of PWV determination), compared with the patients with a smaller number of risk factors and events. This inverse relationship between presumed atherosclerotic load and aortic compliance, if confirmed by prospective studies, may lead to the use of such measurement as a noninvasive marker of vascular risk. More recently, Blacher et al. [10] investigated a cohort of essential hypertensive patients with or without atherosclerosis alterations defined on the basis of clinical events. Their results showed higher carotid-femoral PWV (aortic) in the presence of atherosclerosis alterations even after adjustments on confounding factors. They found that aortic PWV determined from a single measurement is the first determinant of the extent of atherosclerosis assessed as the sum of the atherosclerotic sites. The odds ratios of atherosclerosis alterations according to prognostic variables are shown in *table I*. The optimal cut-off value of PWV as a diagnostic test to detect the presence of atherosclerosis alterations is 13 m/s.

Pulse wave velocity as a marker of morbidity and mortality

In order to evaluate the use of epidemiological data to predict the occurrence of arteriosclerotic diseases, Suzuki [11] investigated from 1983 to 1986 more than 100 thousand Japanese urban residents in whom various examinations including aortic PWV were performed. During the two-year follow-up period, 301 cardiac and cerebrovascular events occurred. Analysis of the results showed that the occurrence of these diseases could not have been predicted from any one specific abnormal result on a screening test, but might have been predicted from multiple abnormal results including PWV. The author suggested that such evaluation may be used to predict the onset of arteriosclerotic diseases to some degree and can contribute to preventive medicine.

TABLE I. Odds ratios of atherosclerotic alterations according to prognostic variables
in hypertensive patients. Data were adjusted on all the presented variables.
(Adapted from Blacher et al. [10].)

Prognostic variable	Adjusted odds ratio (95%CI)
Plasma creatinine (μmol/L)	
< 70*	1.00
70–90	1.80 (0.89–3.63)
90–110	1.42 (0.99–2.04)
> 110	1.70 (1.31–2.21)
Tobacco lifelong dose (pack-years)	
0*	1.00
0–20	1.54 (0.89–2.66)
> 20	1.93 (1.54–2.42)
Age (years)	
< 50*	1.00
50–60	1.50 (0.75–3.05)
60–70	1.49 (1.01–2.18)
> 70	1.57 (1.20–2.06)
PWV (m/s)	
< 10.5*	1.00
10.5–12	1.14 (0.57–2.26)
12–15	1.08 (0.76–1.24)
> 15	1.34 (1.03–1.76)
Diastolic blood pressure (mmHg)	
< 70*	1.00
70–90	0.69 (0.43–1.11)
90–110	0.83 (0.62–1.12)
> 110	0.75 (0.56–0.98)
Diabetes mellitus (yes, no)	
No*	1.00
Yes	1.62 (0.98–2.68)

* Category served as reference group.

Blacher et al. [10] investigated a cohort of essential hypertensive patients with or without atherosclerosis alterations and analysed aortic PWV as a marker of cardio-vascular risk on the basis of Framingham equations. Their results showed a constant increase in carotid femoral PWV values with all the fatal and non-fatal risk events calculation: MI, CHD, CVD and stroke *(figure 2)*. The odds ratios of being in a high-risk group according to the presence versus absence of cardiovascular risk factors are shown in *table II*. Aortic PWV appeared as a stronger predictor than plasma creatinine, LV hypertrophy and total/HDL cholesterol for any type of cardiovascular risk. Further-more, at any given age, aortic PWV was the best predictor of cardiovascular mortality. The optimal cut-off value of PWV, as a diagnostic test, in order to detect ten-year cardiovascular mortality high-risk patients was 13 m/s. These results show that carotid-femoral PWV is strongly associated with the presence and extent of atherosclerosis, and constitutes a forceful marker and predictor of cardiovascular risk in hypertensive patients.

Lehmann et al. [8] have reported results of interim analysis of an ongoing prospective longitudinal follow-up study in non-insulin dependent diabetics (NIDD). Patients who have since died had significantly stiffer aortas at baseline than NIDD patients who are

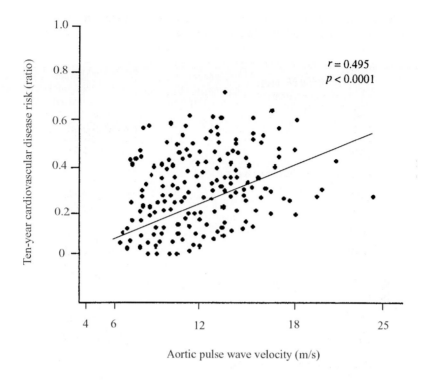

FIGURE 2. Relationship between ten-year cardiovascular risk and carotid-femoral pulse wave velocity in hypertensive patients. (Adapted from Blacher et al. [10].)

still alive and non-diabetic controls matched on age, gender, smoking and treatment status. If the full longitudinal follow-up study confirms these results, measurement of aortic compliance using PWV determination may permit the early identification of NIDD patients at increased risk of vascular complications and death in later life.

Impact of aortic stiffness, as evaluated by carotid-femoral PWV, on survival in end-stage renal disease has recently been evaluated [12]. On the basis of the Cox analysis, two factors emerged as predictors of all-cause and cardiovascular mortality: age, and aortic PWV. After adjustment for all confounding factors, PWV was the strongest predictor of mortality, followed by the duration of hemodialysis. The odds ratio for PWV > 12.0 versus 9.4 m/s was 5.4 (95% CI, 2.4 to 11.9) for all-cause mortality and 5.9 (95% CI, 2.3 to 15.5) for cardiovascular mortality. For each PWV increase of 1 m/s, the all-cause mortality-adjusted odds ratio was 1.39 (95% CI, 1.19 to 1.62) *(table III)*. These results show that in patients with end-stage renal disease, increased aortic stiffness, assessed by measurement of carotid-femoral PWV, is a strong independent predictor of all-cause and mainly cardiovascular mortality *(figure 3)*. In addition, aortic PWV measurements could serve as an important tool in identifying patients at high risk.

In summary, the evaluation of the prognostic value of PWV shows:

– significant correlations and powerful interactions between PWV and both the major and the minor cardiovascular risk factors observed in different populations;

TABLE II. Odds ratios of being in the high-risk group according to the presence versus absence of cardiovascular risk factors in hypertensive patients. (Adapted from Blacher et al. [10].)

Parameter	Odds ratio				
	Coronary heart disease	Coronary heart disease mortality	Stroke	Cardio-vascular disease	Cardio-vascular mortality
PWV (> 13.5 m/s)	4.6	4.9	6.1	5.3	7.1
Sex (male)	7.1	7.3	2.0	3.8	2.9
Age (> 60 years)	3.9	7.3	11.1	6.1	12.9
Plasma glucose (> 7.0 mmol/L)	5.9	5.5	7.1	8.4	4.7
Hypertension (> 160/90 mmHg)	3.4	3.2	6.8	3.6	2.8
Current smoker (yes–no)	3.7	2.6	1.9	3.8	2.2
Tobacco lifelong dose (> 20 pack/years)	2.0	1.9	1.7	2.6	1.7
Total/HDL cholesterol (ratio > 5)	3.9	3.6	1.5	3.6	2.8
LV hypertrophy (yes–no)	11.2	3.0	2.2	4.9	4.5
Plasma creatinine (>100 μmol/L)	2.5	2.7	1.7	1.8	1.8

– significant correlations between PWV and different indicators of arterial atherosclerosis;

– significant correlations between PWV and organ damage, such as microalbuminuria, left ventricular hypertrophy and arterial alterations;

– PWV constitutes a marker of atherosclerosis in different populations. In hypertensive patients, an optimal value of carotid-femoral PWV of 13 m/s, as a diagnostic test to detect the presence of atherosclerosis, has been reported;

– PWV has been reported in hypertensive patients as a strong predictor for any type of cardiovascular risks, and as the best predictor of cardiovascular mortality at any given age;

– interim analysis of an ongoing longitudinal study in NIDD patients showed stiffer aortas at baseline in patients who had died than in those who were still alive;

– PWV is a strong and independent predictor of all-cause and cardiovascular mortality in patients with end-stage renal disease undergoing hemodialysis.

TABLE III. Odds ratio of all-cause and cardiovascular mortality according to prognostic variables divided into tertiles in patients undergoing hemodialysis. (Adapted from Blacher et al. [12].)

Prognostic variable	All-cause mortality		Cardiovascular mortality	
	Deaths (n = 73)	Adjusted OR (95% CI)	Deaths (n = 48)	Adjusted OR (95% CI)
PWV (m/s)				
< 9.4*	6	1.0	2	1.0
9.4–12.0	16	2.5 (0.7–9.1)	12	4.2 (0.7–24.5)
> 12.0	51	5.4 (2.4–11.9)	34	5.9 (2.3–15.5)
Age (year)				
< 45*	5	1.0	4	1.0
45–60	27	4.4 (1.2–16.1)	16	2.6 (0.6–10.9)
> 60	41	2.2 (1.1–4.6)	28	1.5 (0.7–3.0)
Hemoglobin (mmol/L)				
< 5.1*	28	1.0	15	1.0
5.1–6.2	22	0.3 (0.1–0.8)	15	0.7 (0.3–1.8)
> 6.2	23	0.6 (0.4–1.0)	18	1.0 (0.6–1.6)
DBP (mmHg)				
< 78*	30	1.0	20	1.0
78–94	23	0.5 (0.2–1.3)	13	0.6 (0.2–1.5)
> 94	20	0.6 (0.3–1.0)	15	0.9 (0.5–1.5)
Time on dialysis before inclusion (month)				
< 12*	16	1.0	10	1.0
12–50	23	1.1 (0.5–2.9)	15	1.1 (0.4–2.8)
> 50	34	2.8 (1.7–4.7)	23	2.2 (1.3–3.6)

* Category served as reference group.

Thus, a certain amount of evidence of the positive prognostic value of PWV has been published; additional outcomes from ongoing retrospective and prospective studies will soon be available. Whether or not the reduction of PWV improves the prognosis for our patients needs to be confirmed by specific prospective studies.

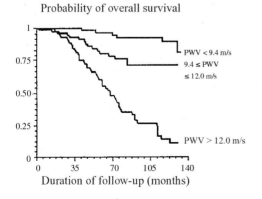
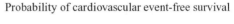
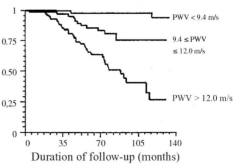

FIGURE 3. Probabilities of overall and event-free survival according to the pulse wave velocity divided in tertiles in patients undergoing hemodialysis. (Adapted from Blacher et al. [12].)

REFERENCES

1 Takegoshi T, Hirai J, Shimada T, Saga T, Kitoh C. The correlation between pulse wave velocity and diabetic angiopathy. Nippon Ronen Igakkai Zasshi 1991 ; 28 : 664-7.

2 Taniwaki H, Nishizawa Y, Kawagishi T, Ishimura E, Emoto M, Okamura T, et al. Decrease in glomerular filtration rate in Japanese patients with type 2 diabetes is linked to atherosclerosis. Diabetes Care 1998 ; 21 : 1848-55.

3 Bouthier JD, De Luca N, Safar ME, Simon AC. Cardiac hypertrophy and arterial distensibility in essential hypertension. Am Heart J 1985 ; 109 : 1345-52.

4 Guarini P, Tedeschi C, Giordano G, Messina V, Cicatiello AM, Strollo L. Effects of hypertension on intimal-medial thickness, left ventricular mass and aortic distensibility. Int Angiol 1994 ; 13 : 317-22.

5 London GM, Guerin AP, Marchais SJ, Pannier B, Safar ME, Day M, et al. Cardiac and arterial interactions in end-stage renal disease. Kidney Int 1996 ; 50 : 600-8.

6 Roman MJ, Pickering TG, Pini R, Schwartz JE, Devereux RB. Prevalence and determinants of cardiac and vascular hypertrophy in hypertension. Hypertension 1995 ; 26 : 369-73.

7 Van Popele N, Grobbee DE, Bots ML, Asmar R, Topouchian J, Hofman A, et al. Association between atherosclerosis and arterial stiffness in an elderly population. 17th Scientific Meeting of the International Society of Hypertension, Workgroup on Arterial Structure and Function, Amsterdam; 1998.

8 Lehmann ED, Cruickshank JK, Wright JS, Ross JR, Sharp P, Gosling RG. A prospective, longitudinal follow-up study of non-invasive Doppler ultrasound measurements of aortic compliance in non-insulin dependent diabetic patients. Workshop on Arterial Structure and Function, Versailles, France; January 1998.

9 Lehmann ED, Hopkins KD, Rawesh A, Joseph RC, Kongoala K, Coppack SW, et al. Relation between number of cardiovascular risk factors/event and noninvasive Doppler ultrasound assessments of aortic compliance. Hypertension 1998 ; 32 : 565-9.

10 Blacher J, Asmar R, Djane S, London GM, Safar ME. Aortic pulse wave velocity as a marker of cardiovascular risk in hypertensive patients. Hypertension 1999 ; 33 : 1111-7.

11 Suzuki K. Use of epidemiological data to predict the occurrence of arteriosclerotic diseases in urban residents. Nippon Ronen Igakkai Zasshi 1996 ; 33 : 360-70.

12 Blacher J, Guérin AP, Pannier B, Marchais SJ, Safar ME, London GM. Impact of aortic stiffness on survival in end-stage renal disease. Circulation 1999 ; 99 : 2434-9.

CHAPTER

Pulse wave velocity and therapy

PULSE WAVE VELOCITY AND DRUG THERAPY

The previous chapters reported that alterations in the mechanical properties of the arterial wall may be observed at an early stage of several cardiovascular diseases or risk factors. The relationships between arterial stiffness and the pathophysiology of these diseases involve complex mechanical and biochemical mechanisms. The observed arterial modifications have been described in various populations as an independent factor of target organ damage and a predictor of cardiovascular morbidity as well as cardiovascular or all-cause mortality. Taken together, these elements highlight the need to evaluate the effects of treatment, not only on the observed risk factor or disease (e.g., high blood pressure) but also on the arterial wall by assessment of its arterial effects. In fact, the arterial wall constitutes the target of all the cardiovascular risk factors and the site of their complications; hence, it is important to assess the ability of the treatment to reverse or improve the arterial abnormalities. This evaluation of the arterial effects of cardiovascular treatment, mainly antihypertensive drugs, is now suggested or even recommended by several authorities. Because of the cyclic stress related to blood pressure variations and because blood pressure is one of the major determinants of arterial stiffness, most of the pharmacological studies performed in this field involve antihypertensive drugs.

Antihypertensive agents and pulse wave velocity

Numerous pharmacological studies have analysed the arterial effects of the different classes of antihypertensives *(table I)*. Some of them have been performed using open protocols or in a single-blind fashion, whereas others were randomized in a double-blind design. Since arterial hypertension affects the arterial system in a different manner, with varied abnormalities at the different arterial sites, it is important to consider the arterial effects of antihypertensive agents according to the arterial site *(figure 1)*. Moreover, it is likely that the response of large arteries to antihypertensive compounds differs according to the specific mechanism of action of each agent. Since different mechanisms may

TABLE I. Pulse wave velocity and antihypertensive therapy.

	Author	Study design	Population	Treatment	Duration	Evaluation criteria	Results	Comments
1	Bouthier 1985	Open	HT	Cadralazine 20 mg Nitrendipine 20 mg	Acute	C-F PWV	BP ↘ with both HR ↗ with Cadralazine PWV ↗ with Nitrendipine PWV ↘ with Cadralazine	For similar BP reduction, different effects on PWV
2	Asmar 1987	Open	HT	Bisoprolol 10 mg OD	4 weeks	B-R PWV	PWV ↘	Evaluation 24 hours after the last dose
3	Asmar 1988	Open	HT	Perindopril 4–8 mg OD	1 year	B-R PWV	PWV ↘	Patients had normalised BP
4	Asmar 1988	Open placebo-controlled	HT	Perindopril 4–8 mg OD	12 weeks	B-R PWV	PWV ↘	After cessation of treatment, PWV ↗
5	Safar 1988	Open placebo-controlled	HT	Indapamide 2.5 mg OD	12 weeks	B-R PWV	PWV ≡	Improvement of systemic compliance. Not significant at the brachial artery
6	Kelly 1989	DB	HT	Dilevalol 200–400 mg OD Atenolol 50–150 mg OD	12 weeks	PWV Aorta-Arm Leg	PWV ↘ in the 3 regions with both drugs versus placebo	PWV reduction related to BP decrease
7	Lacolley 1989	DB	HT	Captopril 75 mg Cadralazine 20 mg	Acute	C-F PWV	PWV ↘ with Captopril PWV ≡ with Cadralazine	For similar BP reduction, different arterial effects
8	Levenson 1989	Open	HT	Nicorandil 20 mg	Acute	B-R PWV	PWV ↘	Decrease in BP
9	Pancera 1989	DB	HT	Lacidipine 4 mg OD Nifédipine 20 mg BD	6 months	B-R PWV	PWV ↘	Increase in compliance based on PWV
10	Benetos 1990	Open	HT	Dihydralazine 4 µg·kg⁻¹·min⁻¹ Perindoprilat 1 and 2.5 µg·kg⁻¹·min⁻¹	Acute	C-F PWV	PWV ↘ in high dose Perindoprilat	Significant increase in heart rate with Dihydralazine

TABLE I. (continued).

	Author	Study design	Population	Treatment	Duration	Evaluation criteria	Results	Comments
11	Laurent 1990	Open	HT	Indapamide 2.5 mg OD Canreonate 50 mg OD	6 weeks	B-R PWV	PWV ≡	Unchanged PWV despite BP reduction
12	Asmar 1991	DB	HT	Bisoprolol 10 mg OD	4 weeks	C-F ; B-R ; F-T PWV	C-F ; B-R PWV ↗ F-T ≡	Decrease in PWV and BP. F-T PWV ↗ but NS
13	Benetos 1991	Open	HT	Ramipril 5 mg	6 weeks	C-F ; B-R ; F-T PWV	C-F ↗ ; F-T ; B-R ≡	Correlation between BP and PWV reduction
14	Asmar 1992	DB	HT	Trandolapril 2, 4 or 8 mg OD	1 week	C-F PWV	PWV ↗ correlation between dose and PW changes	No significant correlation between changes in PWV and BP
15	Asmar 1992	DB	HT	Nitrendipine 20 mg OD	4 weeks	C-F ; B-R ; F-T PWV	C-F ↗ ; F-T ; B-R ≡	No significant correlation between changes in BP and PWV
16	De Cesaris 1992	Open	HT	Nicardipine 40 mg BD Atenolol 100 mg OD	8 months	B-R PWV	PWV ≡ Atenolol PWV ↗ Nicardipine	Different effects on PWV for similar BP reduction
17	Asmar 1992	DB	HT	Lisinopril 5, 10, 20 mg	Acute	C-F ; F-T PWV	C-F and F-T PWV ↗ at the dose of 20 mg	F-T PWV was markedly influenced by the drug dose
18	Asmar 1993	DB	HT	Felodipine 5–10 mg OD Hydrochlorothiazide 25–50 mg OD	6 weeks	C-F, B-R, F-T PWV	PWV ≡ HCTZ PWV ↗ Felodipine	Slight higher decrease in systolic BP with Felodipine
19	De Cesaris 1993	Open	HT	Metoprolol 200 mg OD Lisinopril 20 mg OD	10 months	B-R PWV	PWV ↗ Lisinopril PWV ≡ Metoprolol	Different effect on PWV for similar BP reduction
20	Tedeschi 1993	Open	HT	Nicardipine 40 mg BD	6 months	C-F PWV	PWV ↗	No control group
21	Barenbrock 1994	DB	HT	Lisinopril : 5, 10 or 20 mg OD Metoprolol 50, 100, 200 mg OD	10 weeks	Ultrasound carotid distensibility	Distensibility ↗ in Lisinopril but not in Metoprolol group	Different arterial effects for similar BP reduction
22	Simon 1994	DB	HT	Isradipine 2.5–5 mg OD Metoprolol 50–100 mg OD	3 months	B-R PWV	PWV ↗ Isradipine PWV ≡ Metoprolol	Different arterial effects for similar BP reduction

TABLE I. (continued).

	Author	Study design	Population	Treatment	Duration	Evaluation criteria	Results	Comments
23	Kool 1995	DB	HT	Perindopril 4 mg OD Amlor 2.5/25 HCTZ OD	6 months	Ultrasound carotid distensibility	Distensibility ↗ Perindopril Distensibility ≡ Diuretics	Different arterial effects
24	Pannier 1994	DB	HT	Lacidipine 2 mg	Acute	C-F PWV	PWV ≡ Lacidipine PWV ≡ placebo	Despite the BP reduction no changes in PWV
25	Savolainen 1996	DB	HT	Cilazapril 5 mg OD Atenolol 100 mg OD	6 months	Ascending aorta stiffness MRI	Improvement of elastic modulus with both drugs	Similar changes with both drugs
26	Benetos 1996	DB	HT	HCTZ +Amiloride 50 mg/5 mg OD HCTZ + Captopril 25/50 mg OD	3 months	Ultrasound carotid-aorta	Increased aortic distensibility with both drugs. Carotid distensibility ≡	Similar BP reduction. Different effects according to the site
27	Benetos 1996	Open	HT	Perindopril 4 mg OD Nitrendipine 10–20 mg OD	2 months	C-F PWV	Higher decrease in PWV with Perindopril in the AC + CC groups	AT1R receptor gene polymorphism influences the arterial effects
28	Kahonen 1998	DB	Healthy volunteers	Captopril 25 mg Propranolol 40 mg Verapamil 80 mg	Acute	Aorto-popliteal PWV	Captopril ↗ PWV Propranolol ↗ PWV Isoptine ≡ PWV	Healthy volunteers
29	Breithaupt-Grögler 1998	Randomised DB ?	HT	Verapamil + Trandolapril 180/1 mg OD Metoprolol + HCTZ 100/12.5 mg OD	6 months	C-F PWV	PWV decreased to higher extent with Verapamil + Trandolapril	More pronounced BP reduction with Verapamil + Trandolapril
30	Topouchian 1998	DB	HT	Quinapril 20 mg	Acute	C-F; C-R PWV	PWV ↗ Effects differ according to the site	Maximal effects on muscular arteries
31	Topouchian 1999	DB	HT	Verapamil 240 mg OD Trandolapril 2 mg OD Trandolapril / Verapamil 2 mg/180 mg OD	6 months	C-F PWV	Similar decrease of PWV with the 3 treatments	Changes in distensibility showed significant site effects

DB: double-blind; HT: hypertensives; C-F: carotid-femoral; B-R: brachial-radial. F-T: femoral-tibial: AC and CC relate to polymorphisms of the AT₁ receptors.

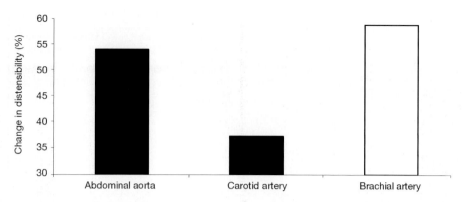

FIGURE 1. Relative change in distensibility after antihypertensive treatment in three arterial territories: abdominal aorta, carotid artery and brachial artery. (Adapted from Topouchian et al. [31].) A significant site effect was noticed.

be involved in the possible improvement of the structural and functional properties under treatment, the arterial effects of the antihypertensive agents have to be considered in short-term but also, and principally, in long-term treatment. Finally, since the arterial effect of an antihypertensive compound may not necessarily be related to its antihypertensive effect, several doses have to be analysed. Therefore, evaluation of the arterial effects of an antihypertensive agent must consider the arterial site on which measurements are performed, the doses used, and the duration of the treatment.

Table II shows most of the open or single-blind pharmacological studies based on PWV to evaluate the arterial effects of antihypertensive treatments.

Results of acute administration or a short-term treatment period (< 28 days) showed no significant effect on aortic PWV with vasodilators such as cadralazine or dihydralazine, and a decrease in brachial-radial PWV with nicorandil. Lower aortic PWV (higher distensibility) has been observed in one study for nitrendipine and one study with perindopril.

During long-term treatment (≥ 28 days) most of the beta-blockers (except bisoprolol) showed no significant modifications at the limb level. For the calcium antagonists, nicardipine showed a decrease in aortic and brachial-radial PWV. Concerning the ACE-inhibitors, most of the studies exhibited a significant decrease of PWV measured at the aortic and the arm levels. Diuretics did not show significant changes.

Therefore, according to these results, diuretics, vasodilators (except nicorandil) and beta-blockers (except bisoprolol) did not induce significant changes in PWV. Calcium antagonists and principally ACE-inhibitors exhibited significant improvement of PWV at the aortic and the brachial levels.

Table III shows most of the double-blind pharmacological studies based on PWV measurements to evaluate the arterial effects of several antihypertensive agents. Few studies have been performed using an acute administration or short-term treatment period; most of them included various ACE-inhibitors with improvement of PWV. During long-term treatment, diuretics showed no significant effects, beta-blockers exhibited variable results according to the drug used, a constant increase in arterial distensibility

TABLE II. PWV changes observed in open or single-blind studies with antihypertensive agents.

		Acute and short-term treatment < 28 days		Long-term treatment ≥ 28 days	
		Aorta	Arm/Leg	Aorta	Arm/Leg
Vasodilators & equivalent					
• Bouthier [1]	Cadralazine	unchanged			
• Levenson [8]	Nicorandil		↘		
• Benetos [10]	Dihydralazine	unchanged			
Beta-blockers					
• De Cesaris [16]	Atenolol				unchanged
• Asmar[2]	Bisoprolol			↘	
• De Cesaris [19]	Metoprolol				unchanged
Calcium-antagonists					
• Bouthier [1]	Nitrendipine	↘			
• De Cesaris [16]	Nicardipine				↘
• Tedeschi [20]	Nitrendipine			↘	
• Benetos [13]	Nicardipine			(↘)	
ACE-inhibitors					
• Asmar [3, 4]	Perindopril				↘
• Benetos [10]	Perindopril	↘			
• Benetos [13]	Ramipril			↘	unchanged
• De Cesaris [19]	Lisinopril				↘
• Benetos [27]	Perindopril			↘	
Diuretics					
• Laurent [11]	Canreanate				unchanged
	Indapamide				
• Safar [5]	Indapamide				unchanged

was observed with ACE-inhibitors, and less marked improvement was reported with calcium antagonists.

Recently, Delerme et al. [32] took advantage of several pharmacological studies conducted between 1987 and 1994 under similar methodological conditions and performed a meta-analysis on individual data. Only controlled randomized double-blind parallel-group trials analyzing the effects of various antihypertensive agents or placebos on carotid-femoral PWV either during short-term (< 28 days) or long-term (≥ 28 days) were selected. The results showed that in short- and long-term trials, antihypertensive agents reduced PWV by comparison to placebos independently of blood pressure reduction and after adjustment on baseline parameters. The pressure-independent decrease in PWV was more pronounced with chronic than with acute or short-term treatment. This improvement of PWV was more pronounced after ACE-inhibitors than after calcium-antagonists in short-term trials, and after ACE-inhibitors, beta-blockers or diuretics than after calcium-antagonists in long-term trials. The results of this meta-analysis suggest higher efficacy of ACE-inhibitors on aortic PWV. Nevertheless, it is important to note here that limited different compounds were included in each antihypertensive class. In fact, beta-blockers included only bisoprolol, which has been shown to exhibit significant changes of PWV by comparison to the other beta-blockers. Therefore, before extrapolating the results observed with one specific antihypertensive agent to other agents of its class and making hasty conclusions about a 'class-effect', more specific studies performed in large populations are needed (*table IV, figures 2, 3, 4*).

TABLE III. PWV changes observed in double-blind studies with antihypertensive treatment.

		Acute and short-term treatment < 28 days		Long-term treatment ≥ 28 days	
		Aorta	Arm/Leg	Aorta	Arm/Leg
Vasodilators					
• Lacolley [7]	Cadralazine	unchanged			
Beta-blockers					
• Kelly [6]	Dilevalol			↘	↘
	Atenolol			↘	↘
• Asmar [12]	Bisoprolol			↘	↘/≡
• Barenbrock [21]	Metoprolol			unchanged (carotid)	
• Simon [22]	Metoprolol				unchanged
• Savolainen [25]	Atenolol			improvement (MRI)	
• Kahonen [28]	Propranolol	↘ (normotensive)			
Calcium antagonists					
• Pancera [9]	Lacidipine				↘
	Nifedipine				↘
• Asmar [15]	Nitrendipine			↘	unchanged
• Asmar [18]	Felodipine			↘	↘
• Simon [22]	Isradipine				↘
• Pannier [24]	Lacidipine	unchanged			
• Kahonen [28]	Verapamil	↘ (normotensive)			
• Topouchian [31]	Verapamil			↘	
ACE-Inhibitors					
• Lacolley [7]	Captopril	↘			
• Asmar [14]	Trandolapril	↘			
• Asmar [17]	Lisinopril	↘	↘		
• Barenbrock [21]	Lisinopril			distensibility ↗ (carotid)	
• Kool [23]	Perindopril			distensibility ↗ (carotid)	
• Savolainen [25]	Cilazapril			improvement (aorta-MRI)	
• Benetos [26]	Perindopril			↘	
• Kahonen [28]	Captopril	↘ (normotensive)			
• Topouchian [30]	Quinapril	↘	↘		
• Topouchian [31]	Trandolapril			↘	
Diuretics					
• Asmar [18]	Hydrochlorothiazide (HCTZ)			unchanged	unchanged
• Kool [23]	Amiloride + HCTZ			unchanged (carotid)	
• Benetos [26]	Amiloride + HCTZ			↘	

Large-population clinical trials

In order to analyse whether long-term antihypertensive treatment can fully reverse arterial alterations in treated hypertensives with normalized diastolic BP, we measured carotid-femoral PWV in normotensives, untreated hypertensives and a cohort of treated hypertensives [33]. The latter included hypertensive patients aged from 27 to 81 years, all of them treated and classified as well-controlled by antihypertensive treatment (what-

TABLE IV. Changes in blood pressure and PWV after felodipine and hydrochlorothiazide in hypertensive patients. (Adapted from Asmar et al. [18].)

	Baseline	Felodipine	Hydrochlorothiazide
Systolic blood pressure (mmHg)	166 ± 15	142 ± 16	150 ± 15*
Diastolic blood pressure (mmHg)	102 ± 5	88 ± 9	91 ± 8
Carotid-femoral PWV (m/s)	10.9 ± 2.0	9.2 ± 1.8	10.1 ± 2**
Femoral-tibial PWV (m/s)	12.8 ± 1.7	11.1 ± 1.9	12.2 ± 1.7**
Carotid-radial PWV (m/s)	11.7 ± 1.9	10.0 ± 2	11.8 ± 1.8**

± SD; * $p < 0.05$; ** $p < 0.01$.

ever their treatment) if their diastolic blood pressure < 90 mmHg during the three months preceding the study. The mean duration of the hypertensive disease was 5.6 ± 4.8 years; the mean duration of normalized diastolic BP was 3.9 ± 4.1 years. At the time of the study, 37% of the patients were treated by monotherapy, 32% by bitherapy and 31% by tri- or multiple therapy. All the antihypertensive drug classes were used without significant preponderance. The results showed that when compared with untreated hypertensives, treated hypertensives with well-controlled diastolic BP had significantly lower blood pressure and PWV according to age. However, although diastolic blood pressure of well-controlled hypertensives was not significantly different from that of normotensive subjects, the aortic distensibility of the controlled hypertensives showed a faster increase in PWV with age *(figure 5)*.

To analyse the role of controlling systolic blood pressure on PWV, treated patients were divided into two subgroups: subgroup A, where both diastolic and systolic blood pressure were controlled (< 140/90 mmHg), and subgroup B, where diastolic blood pressure was controlled (< 90 mmHg) but not systolic blood pressure (> 140 mmHg)

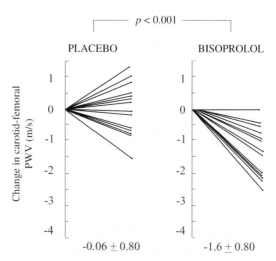

FIGURE 2. Changes in carotid-femoral PWV after one month of treatment with placebo or bisoprolol. (Adapted from Asmar et al. [12].)

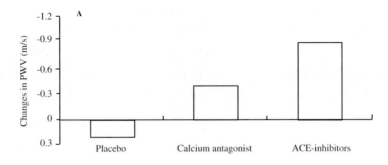

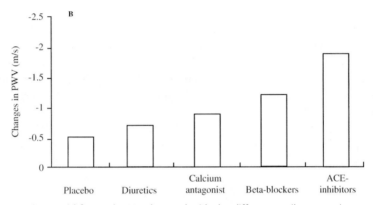

FIGURE 3. Changes in carotid-femoral PWV observed with the different antihypertensive agents from the studies considered in the meta-analysis. (Adapted from Delerme [32].) A. Acute and short-term drug administration (< 28 d). B. Long-term drug administration (≥ 28 d).

(figure 6). The results showed higher PWV in subgroup B, and despite the blood pressure normalization, some patients continued to present PWV values outside the normotensive nomogram. These results suggest that the exclusive choice of diastolic blood pressure as a marker for the vascular complications of hypertension may not be fully adequate, and that specific longitudinal studies are needed to evaluate the ability of antihypertensive drugs to reverse arterial abnormalities.

The Complior® study

The Complior® study is the first large-population clinical trial designed to evaluate the ability of an antihypertensive therapy based on ACE inhibition to improve the arterial abnormalities observed in hypertension [34]. Patients were treated for six months, starting with perindopril 4 mg OD which was increased to 8 mg OD, and combined with a diuretic (indapamide 2.5 mg OD) if blood pressure was uncontrolled (> 140/90 mmHg). Arterial stiffness was assessed at inclusion, and at two and six months after treatment, by carotid-femoral PWV measurements, using the Complior® device. Data collected from 69 centers (19 countries) concerned more than 2,000 patients. The results showed significant ($p < 0.001$) decreases from baseline in blood pressure (systolic: -23.7 ± 16.8, diastolic: -14.6 ± 10 mmHg), and PWV (-1.1 ± 1.4 m/s). Despite a significant

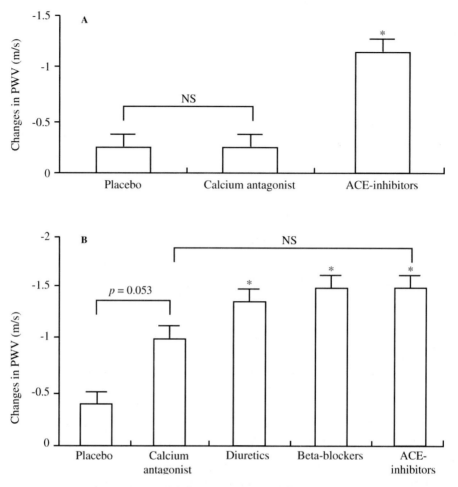

FIGURE 4. Changes in carotid-femoral PWV (adjusted for BP reduction and baseline values). (Adapted from Delerme [32].) A. Acute and short-term drug administration (< 28 d). B. Long-term drug administration (≥ 28 d). *p* < 0.05; NS: non significant.

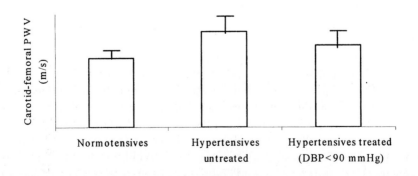

FIGURE 5. Carotid-femoral PWV in normotensives, untreated and treated hypertensives. (Adapted from Asmar et al. [33].)

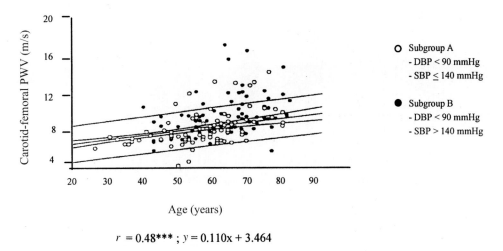

$$r = 0.48*** \; ; \; y = 0.110x + 3.464$$

FIGURE 6. Carotid-femoral PWV (y): relationship with age (x) in well-controlled hypertensive subjects plotted on the normotensive nomogram and its individual and mean 95% confidence limits. (Adapted from Asmar et al. [33].)

TABLE V. Blood pressure and carotid-femoral PWV, mean values and changes from baseline (M0) after a six month treatment (M6). Data from the Complior® study. (Adapted from Asmar et al. [34].)

Variables	M0	M6	Δ M6–M0	p
SBP (mmHg)	158 ± 15	134 ± 13	− 24 – 17	< 0.001
DBP (mmHg)	98 ± 7	84 ± 8	− 14 ± 10	< 0.001
MBP (mmHg)	118 ± 8	100 ± 9	− 18 ± 11	< 0.001
PP (mmHg)	59 ± 15	50 ± 10	− 9 ± 15	< 0.001
HR (bpm)	75 ± 10	75 ± 10	− 0.3 ± 10	NS
PWV (m/s)	11.6 ± 2.6	10.5 ± 2.1	− 1.1 ± 1.4	< 0.001

correlation ($p < 0.001$) between changes in SBP and PWV, less than 10% ($r^2 = 0.06$) of the observed arterial effects were related to blood pressure reduction. Individual analysis showed that PWV improvement was not always concomitant with blood pressure reduction, and vice versa, suggesting a specific arterial effect of the study drug regimen. This study showed that arterial abnormalities observed in hypertension can be reversed by an antihypertensive treatment regimen based on ACE inhibition through mechanisms which are partly independent of blood pressure reduction. Whether this reversal can improve the cardiovascular prognosis of patients needs to be confirmed (*table V, figure 7*).

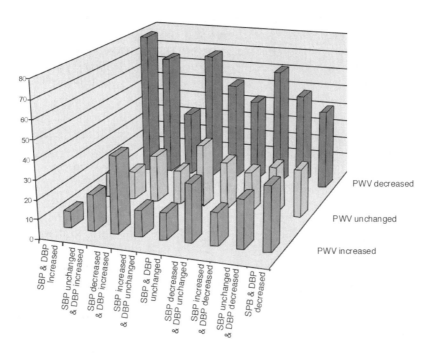

FIGURE 7. Distribution of PWV variations (%) in relation to changes in DBP and SBP. Data from the Complior® study. (Adapted from Asmar et al. [34].)

Arterial stiffness and hormone replacement therapy

Premenopausal women are known to be protected from cardiovascular disease; this protection has been attributed to the effects of sex hormones, principally oestrogen, which may have an effect on the biophysical properties of the arterial wall. In this regard, several studies have analysed the effects of hormone replacement therapy (HRT) on arterial stiffness.

Lehmann et al. [35] assessed aortic compliance on the basis of PWV in healthy postmenopausal women receiving tibolone, a synthetic steroid structurally related to norethisterone, for at least three years. Contrary to their expectations, no significant differences in blood pressure-corrected aortic distensibility were observed between women receiving tibolone and the control group subjects. Elsewhere, Blacher et al. [36] showed that carotid-femoral PWV was slightly higher in women receiving placebos than in those receiving a fixed regimen of estradiol 50/16 TDS patches and 5 mg chlormadinone acetate tablets over four weeks; the difference was not significant (10.27 m/s versus 9.8 m/s). Moreover, Tanaka et al. [37] assessed arterial PWV and carotid augmentation index in healthy postmenopausal women including users and non-users of HRT; no significant differences in any of the physical characteristics of the arterial wall stiffness were noticed between the two groups. In a similar cross-sectional study, Hayword et al. [38] showed that women being administered HRT exhibited no difference in PWV but a lower augmentation index than those not currently receiving HRT, suggesting that HRT may improve the pulsatile vascular afterload.

On the other hand, conflicting results have been reported by numerous authors. In fact, Liang et al. [39] assessed the effects of oestrogen and progesterone on age-related changes in arteries of postmenopausal women. They measured intima-medial thickness and indices of systemic and carotid arterial compliance in groups of older men, postmenopausal women not on HRT and women on long-term HRT with oestrogen alone or oestrogen plus progestin. Carotid intima-medial thickness was reduced in the HRT groups compared with men and the non-HRT group; results for oestrogen and oestrogen plus progestin subgroups were similar. Systemic arterial compliance was higher in both HRT groups compared with the non-HRT group. Indices of carotid stiffness were similar in men and in the non-HRT group. The HRT oestrogen plus progestin group showed increased carotid stiffness compared with the HRT oestrogen group. Their results suggest an apparent protective effect of long-term oestrogen therapy on carotid intima-medial thickness and age-related changes in arterial stiffness, and that progestin may adversely influence arterial stiffness. Elsewhere, Rajkumar et al. [40] assessed total systemic compliance and PWV in premenopausal and postmenopausal women with or without HRT. Arterial compliance was greater in the premenopausal group than in the postmenopausal group not taking hormone therapy. Postmenopausal women taking hormone therapy had a significantly increased systemic arterial compliance compared with women not taking hormone therapy. Aortic PWV was lower in the premenopausal than in the untreated postmenopausal women (6.0 versus 8.9 m/s, $p < 0.001$), and lower in the treated women with HRT than in the untreated women (7.9 versus 8.9 m/s, $p < 0.01$). Moreover, when HRT was withdrawn for four weeks, a significant decrease in systemic arterial compliance and increase in PWV were observed. These results suggest that HRT may decrease stiffness of the aorta and large arteries in postmenopausal women. Similar results were observed in a prospective study performed by Maldonado et al. [41], who showed a significant decrease of carotid-femoral PWV after six months treatment with HRT (11.9 ± 2.9 versus 10.3 ± 2.1 m/s) in post-menopausal women. More recently, the same authors [42] observed similar PWV reduction after a six-month treatment with oral oestrogens and progestins in normotensive women with spontaneous menopause. Furthermore, they observed a significant reduction of carotid-femoral PWV after six months of therapy with transdermic oestrogens (50 μg patch of 17 β estradiol) in normotensive women with surgical menopause [43].

In summary, it appears that HRT may affect arterial distensibility and PWV in a different manner, depending on whether we consider oestrogens or the association of oestrogens and progestins. Prospective and controlled studies are still needed in order to clarify and analyse the pathophysiology of these arterial effects.

Pulse wave velocity and lipid-lowering drugs

Very few studies were performed to evaluate the arterial effects of lipid-lowering drug therapy in patients with primary hyperlipidaemia. Kool et al. [44] reported that carotid, femoral and brachial distensibility were not significantly changed after short-term treatment with pravastatin in patients with primary hypercholesterolemia.

Further studies are needed to evaluate the arterial effects of lipid-lowering drugs in patients with lipid abnormalities.

Pulse wave velocity and anti-diabetic treatments

Studies have shown that microangiopathy is retarded by improving blood glucose control in diabetic patients. Whether or not this is true for macroangiopathy remains unclear. In fact, studies are needed to evaluate the arterial effects of anti-diabetic treatments in both insulin and non-insulin-dependent-diabetics. The few available data [45, 46] suggest that better HbA1C values and glucose control are associated with less stiff carotid arteries. Further studies are needed to evaluate the arterial benefits of the different anti-diabetic treatments.

PULSE WAVE VELOCITY AND NON-PHARMACOLOGICAL THERAPY

(See also chapter IV on Factors influencing PWV.)

Salt intake

Clinical trials and large population studies in a population with low salt intake have shown that PWV measured at three arterial sites (aorta, leg and arm) was consistently lower than in a population with normal or high salt intake. It has been suggested that salt presents an independent effect on arterial tone and arterial wall properties contributing to an increase in arterial stiffness. Moreover, other studies have shown that subjects who followed a low salt diet have reduced arterial stiffness by comparison to that observed in control subjects matched for age and mean blood pressure with a regular diet [47-50]. Similar results were observed in patients with different cardiovascular diseases.

Garlic intake

Studies have suggested that garlic may have protective effects against cardiovascular diseases. Recently, Breithaupt-Grögler et al. [51] investigated healthy adults who were taking ≥ 300 mg/d of standardized garlic powder for ≥ two years by comparison to their age and sex-matched control subjects. Aortic PWV was lower in the garlic group than in the control group. The effect of garlic on PWV was independent of confounding factors. More studies are needed to confirm these observations in populations with cardiovascular diseases and to analyse if such an improvement would persist while using cardiovascular treatments.

Fish oil and fish intake

Comparison of aortic PWV between inhabitants of fishing and farming villages in Japan has shown lower PWV in the fishing villages than in the farming villages. For Hamazaki et al. [52], this is consistent with a lower incidence of ischemic heart disease in the coastal area than in the mountainous area, and these data suggest that a long-term fish diet may slow down sclerotic changes of arteries. Wahlqvist et al. [53] in Australia investigated the relationships between fish consumption and arterial compliance in healthy subjects and in patients with NIDDM. Elsewhere, in a placebo-controlled study, McVeigh et al. [54] investigated the effects of dietary fish oil supplementation on arterial wall characteristics in patients with NIDDM. Their results showed that large artery compliance was improved significantly after six weeks of fish oil therapy. Taken together, these findings support the hypothesis that fish oils favourably influence arterial wall characteristics in healthy subjects and in patients with NIDDM; these direct vascular effects may contribute to the cardioprotective actions of fish oils in humans. More recently, Nestel et al. [55] showed that arterial compliance in obese subjects with markers for insulin resistance is improved with dietary plant n-3 fatty acid from flaxseed oil despite increased LDL oxidizability.

Further controlled studies performed in patients with different cardiovascular diseases are needed to better understand the interactions of the different compounds of fish oils and arterial wall characteristics.

Exercise and physical training

(See also chapter V, section on Pulse wave velocity in athletes.)

Most of the studies performed in endurance athletes and male cyclists have shown lower PWV in sportsmen by comparison to sedentary subjects.

The effect of moderate exercise (treadmill at a speed of 3 mph and 5% grade for 15 minutes) on PWV in normal young men was evaluated by Simonson et al. [56] before and immediately after the exercise; no significant change in the pulse transmission was noticed. Sebban et al. [57] evaluated PWV in elderly women at rest and during exercise; changes in heart rate and oxygen consumption from resting values were strikingly increased, with faster PWV. Reduced arterial distensibility with ageing was found to be the major factor affecting cardiovascular responses to exercise. Murgo et al. [58] showed increased PWV which caused wave reflections to occur earlier during exercise, but the general characteristics of the pressure wave shapes remained unchanged. Siché et al. [59] showed increased PWV values measured at the upper limb level in normotensive and hypertensive patients during exercise. More recently, Kingwell et al. [60] showed reduced aortic and leg PWV 0.5 h post-exercise and suggested that a single bout of cycling exercise increased arterial compliance post-exercise by mechanisms that may relate to vasodilatation.

Taken together, these findings show that regular endurance exercise is associated with lower PWV. Increased PWV was observed during exercise, while in the post-exercise period, a decrease in PWV values was noticed. Further studies are needed to evaluate whether regular endurance exercise improves arterial distensibility in patients with cardiovascular diseases and whether this improvement is independent of cardiovascular treatment.

REFERENCES

1 Bouthier JD, De Luca N, Safar ME, Simon AC. Cardiac hypertrophy and arterial distensibility in essential hypertension. Am Heart J 1985 ; 109 : 1345-52.

2 Asmar R, Hugues C, Pannier B, Daou J, Safar ME. Duration of action of bisoprolol after cessation of a 4 week treatment and its influence on pulse wave velocity and aortic diameter: a pilot study in hypertensive patients. Eur Heart J 1987 ; 8 : 115-20.

3 Asmar R, Journo HJ, Lacolley PJ, Santoni JP, Billaud E, Levy BI, et al. Treatment for one year with perindopril: effect on cardiac mass and arterial compliance in essential hypertension. J Hypertens 1988 ; 6 Suppl 3 : 33-9.

4 Asmar R, Pannier B, Santoni JP, Laurent S, London GM, Levy BI, et al. Reversion of cardiac hypertrophy and reduced arterial compliance after converting enzyme inhibition in essential hypertension. Circulation 1988 ; 78 : 941-50.

5 Safar M, Laurent S, Safavian A, Pannier, Asmar R. Sodium and large arteries in hypertension: effects of indapamide. Am J Med 1988 ; 84 Suppl 1B : 15-9.

6 Kelly R, Daley J, Avolio A, O'Rourke M. Arterial dilation and reduced wave reflection. Hypertension 1989 ; 14 : 14-21.

7 Lacolley PJ, Laurent ST, Billaud EB, Safar ME. Carotid arterial hemodynamics in hypertension: acute administration of captopril or cadralazine. Cardiovas Drug Ther 1989 ; 3 : 859-63.

8 Levenson J, Bouthier J, Chau NP, Roland E, Simon AC. Effects of nicorandil on arterial and venous vessels of the forearm in systemic hypertension. Am J Cardiol 1989 ; 63 : 40J-43J.

9 Pancera P, Arosio E, Arcaro G, Priante F, Montesi G, Paluani F, et al. Haemodynamic parameters in hypertensive patients: changes induced by lacidipine and nifedipine. J Hypertens 1989 ; 7 Suppl 6 : 284-5.

10 Benetos A, Santoni JP, Safar ME. Vascular effects of intravenous infusion of the angiotensin converting enzyme inhibitor perindoprilat. J Hypertens 1990 ; 8 : 819-26.

11 Laurent S, Lacolley PM, Cuche JL, Safar ME. Influence of diuretics on brachial artery diameter and distensibility in hypertensive patients. Fundam Clin Pharmacol 1990 ; 4 : 685-93.

12 Asmar R, Kerihuel JC, Girerd XJ, Safar ME. Effect of bisoprolol on blood pressure and arterial hemodynamics in systemic hypertension. Am J Cardiol 1991 ; 68 : 61-4.

13 Benetos A, Asmar R, Vasmant D, Thiéry P, Safar ME. Long lasting arterial effects of the ACE-inhibitor ramipril. J Hum Hypertens 1991 ; 5 : 363-8.

14 Asmar R, Benetos A, Darne BM, Pauly NC, Safar ME. Converting enzyme inhibition : dissociation between antihypertensive and arterial effects. J Hum Hypertens 1992 ; 6 : 381-5.

15 Asmar R, Benetos A, Brahimi M, Chaouche-Teyara K, Safar M. Arterial and antihypertensive effects of nitrendipine: a double-blind comparison versus placebo. J Cardiovasc Pharmacol 1992 ; 20 : 858-63.

16 De Cesaris R, Ranieri G, Filitti V, Andriani A. Large artery compliance in essential hypertension. Effect of calcium antagonism and β-blocking. Am J Hypertens 1992 ; 5 : 624-8.

17 Asmar R, Iannascoli F, Benetos A, Safar ME. Dose optimization study of arterial changes associated with angiotensin converting enzyme inhibition in hypertension. J Hypertens 1992 ; 10 Suppl 5 : 13-9.

18 Asmar R, Benetos A, Chaouche-Teyara K, Raveau-Landon CM, Safar ME. Comparison of effects of felodipine versus hydrochlorothiazide on arterial diameter and pulse wave velocity in essential hypertension. Am J Cardiol 1993 ; 72 : 794-8.

19 De Cesaris R, Ranieri G, Filitti V, Andriani A, Bonfantino MV. Forearm arterial distensibility in patients with hypertension: comparative effects of long-term ACE inhibition and β-blocking. Clin Pharmacol Ther 1993 ; 53 : 360-7.

20 Tedeschi C, Guarini P, Giodano G, Messina V, Cicatiello AM, Jovino L, et al. Effects of nicardipine on intimal-medial thickness and arterial distensibility in hypertensive patients. Int Angiol 1993 ; 12 : 344-7.

21 Barenbrock M, Speicker C, Hoeks APG, Zidek W, Rahn KH. Effect of lisinopril and metoprolol on arterial distensibility. Hypertension 1994 ; 23 Suppl I : 161-3.

22 Simon A, Merli I, Del Pino M, Bräutigam M, Welzel D, Burger KJ, et al. Vasoselective and drug-specific effects of isradipine on large arterial vessels in hypertensive patients compared to metoprolol. Arzneimittel Forschung 1994 ; 44 : 305-9.

23 Kool MJ, Lustermans FA, Breed JG, Struyker Boudier HA, Hoeks AP, Reneman RS, et al. The influence of perindopril and the diuretic combination amiloride + hydrochlorothiazide on the vessel wall properties of large arteries in hypertensive patients. J Hypertens 1995 ; 13 : 839-48.

24 Pannier BM, Lafeche AB, Girerd X, London GM, Safar ME. Arterial stiffness and wave reflections following acute calcium blockade in essential hypertension. Am J Hypertens 1994 ; 7 : 168-76.

25 Savolainen A, Keto P, Poutanen VP, Hekali P, Standertskjöld-Nordenstam CG, Rames A, et al. Effects of angiotensin-converting enzyme inhibition versus β-adrenergic blockade on aortic stiffness in essential hypertension. J Cardiovasc Pharmacol 1996 ; 27 : 99-104.

26 Benetos A, Lafleche A, Asmar R, Gautier S, Safar A, Safar ME. Arterial stiffness, hydrochlorothiazide and converting enzyme inhibition in essential hypertension. J Hum Hypertens 1996 ; 10 : 77-82.

27 Benetos A, Cambien F, Gautier S, Ricard S, Safar M, Laurent S, et al. Influence of the angiotensin II type 1 receptor gene polymorphism on the effects of perindopril and nitrendipine on arterial stiffness in hypertensive individuals. Hypertension 1996 ; 28 : 1081-4.

28 Kahonen M, Ylitalo R, Koobi T, Turjanmaa V, Ylitalo P. Influence of captopril, propranolol, and verapamil on arterial pulse wave velocity and other cardiovascular parameters in healthy volunteers. Int J Clin Pharmacol Ther 1998 ; 36 : 483-9.

29 Breithaupt-Grögler K, Gerhardt G, Lehmann G, Notter T, Belz GG. Blood pressure and aortic elastic properties-verapamil SR/trandolapril compared to a metoprolol/hydrochlorothiazide combination therapy. Int J Clin Pharmacol Ther 1998 ; 36 : 425-31.

30 Topouchian J, Brisac AM, Pannier B, Vicaut E, Safar M, Asmar R. Assessment of the acute arterial effects of converting enzyme inhibition in essential hypertension: a double-blind, comparative and crossover study. J Hum Hypertens 1998 ; 12 : 181-7.

31 Topouchian J, Asmar R, Sayegh F, Rudnicki A, Benetos A, Bacri AM, et al. Changes in arterial structure and function under trandolapril-verapamil combination in hypertension. Stroke 1999 ; 30 : 1056-64.

32 Delerme S. Amélioration pression-indépendante de la distensibilité des gros troncs artériels par le traitement anti-hypertenseur [DEA de pharmacologie expérimentale et clinique]. Paris : Université Paris XI; 1997-1998.

33 Asmar R, Benetos A, London GM, Hugue C, Weiss Y, Topouchian J, et al. Aortic distensibility in normotensive, untreated and treated hypertensive patients. Blood Pressure 1995 ; 4 : 48-54.

34 Asmar R, Topouchian J, Crisan O, Pannier B, Rudnichi A, Safar M. Reversal of arterial abnormalities by long-term antihypertensive therapy in a large population. The Complior® study. J Hypertens 1999 ; 17 Suppl 3 : S9.

35 Lehmann ED, Hopkins KD, Parker JR, Turay RC, Rymer J, Fogelman I, et al. Aortic distensibility in post-menopausal women receiving Tibolone. Br J Radiol 1994 ; 67 : 701-5.

36 Blacher J, Raison J, Amah G, Schiemann AL, Stimpel M, Safar ME. Increased arterial distensibility in postmenopausal hypertensive women with and without hormone replacement therapy after acute administration of the ACE-inhibitor moexipril. Cardiovasc Drugs Ther 1998 ; 12 : 409-14.

37 Tanaka H, DeSouza CA, Seals DR. Arterial stiffness and hormone replacement use in healthy postmenopausal women. J Gerontol A Biol Sci Med Sci 1998 ; 53 : M344-6.

38 Hayward CS, Knight DC, Wren BG, Kelly RP. Effect of hormone replacement therapy on non-invasive cardiovascular haemodynamics. J Hypertens 1997 ; 15 : 987-93.

39 Liang YL, Teede H, Shiel LM, Thomas A, Craven R, Sachithanandan N, et al. Effects of oestrogen and progesterone on age-related changes in arteries of postmenopausal women. Clin Exp Pharmacol Physiol 1997 ; 24 : 457-9.

40 Rajkumar C, Kingwell BA, Cameron JD, Waddell T, Mehra R, Christophidis N, et al. Hormonal therapy increases arterial compliance in postmenopausal women. J Am Coll Cardiol 1997 ; 30 : 350-6.

41 Maldonado J, Aguas Lopez F, Barbosa A, Alves Z, Pego M, Teixeira F, et al. Circadian blood pressure profile, variability and arterial distensibility in postmenopausal women before and after hormonal replacement therapy. Am J Hypertens 1998 ; 11 : 95A.

42 Maldonado J, Aguas Lopez F, Pego M, Pereira T, Damas P, Alves Z, et al. The association of estrogens and progestins as replacement therapy don't change blood pressure but decrease PWV in normotensive postmenopausal women. Am J Hypertens 1998 ; 11 : 95A.

43 Maldonado J, Aguas Lopez F, Pego M, Peireira T, Alves M, Alves Z, et al. Estrogen replacement therapy does not change blood pressure but decreases PWV in normotensive postmenopausal women. Am J Hypertens 1998 ; 11 : 95A.

44 Kool MJ, Lustermans FA, Kragten H, Struyker Boudier HA, Hoeks AP, Reneman RS, et al. Does lowering of cholesterol levels influence functional properties of large arteries? Eur J Clin Pharmacol 1995 ; 48 : 217-23.

45 Blankenhorn DH, Hodis HN. Atherosclerosis – reversal with therapy. West J Med 1993 ; 159 : 172-9.

46 Jensen-Urstad KJ, Reichard PG, Rosfors JS, Lindblad LE, Jensen-Urstad MT. Early atherosclerosis is retarded by improved long-term blood glucose control in patients with IDDM. Diabetes 1996 ; 45 : 1253-8.

47 Avolio AP, Clyde KM, Beard TC, Cooke HM, Ho KL, O'Rourke MF. Improved arterial distensibility in normotensive subjects on a low salt diet. Arteriosclerosis 1986 ; 6 : 166-9.

48 Safar ME, Asmar R, Benetos A, Levy BI, London GM. Sodium, large arteries, and diuretic compounds in hypertension. Am J Med Sci 1994 ; 307 Suppl 1 : 3-8.

49 Draaijer P, Kool MJ, Maessen JM, Van Bortel LM, de Leeuw PW, Van Hoof JP, et al. Vascular distensibility and compliance in salt-sensitive and salt-resistant borderline hypertension. J Hypertens 1993 ; 11 : 1199-207.

50 Benetos A, Xiao YY, Cuche JL, Hannaert P, Safar M. Arterial effects of salt restriction in hypertensive patients. A 9-week, randomized, double-blind, crossover study. J Hypertens 1992 ; 10 : 355-60.

51 Breithaupt-Grögler K, Ling M, Boudoulas H, Belz GG. Protective effect of chronic garlic intake on elastic properties of aorta in the elderly. Circulation 1997 ; 96 : 2649-55.

52 Hamazaki T, Urakaze M, Sawazaki S, Yamazaki K, Taki H, Yano S. Comparison of pulse wave velocity of the aorta between inhabitants of fishing and farming villages in Japan. Atherosclerosis 1988 ; 73 : 157-60.

53 Wahlqvist ML, Lo CS, Myers KA. Fish intake and arterial wall characteristics in healthy people and diabetic patients. Lancet 1989 ; 2 : 944-6.

54 McVeigh GE, Brennan GM, Cohn JN, Finkelstein SM, Hayes RJ, Johnston GD. Fish oil improves arterial compliance in non-insulin-dependent diabetes mellitus. Arterioscler Thromb 1994 ; 14 : 1425-9.

55 Nestel PJ, Pomeroy SE, Sasahara T, Yamashita T, Liang YL, Dart AM, et al. Arterial compliance in obese subjects is improved with dietary plant n-3 fatty acid from flaxseed oil despite increased LDL oxidizability. Arterioscler Thromb Vasc Biol 1997 ; 17 : 1163-70.

56 Simonson E, Koff S, Keys A, Minckler J. Contour of the toe pulse reactive hyperemia, and pulse transmission velocity : group and repeat variability, effect of age, exercise, and disease. Am Heart J 1955 ; 50 : 260-79.

57 Sebban C, Berthaux P, Lenoir H, Eugene M, Venet R, Memin Y, et al. Arterial compliance, systolic pressure and heart rate in elderly women at rest and on exercise. Gerontology 1981 ; 27 : 271-80.

58 Murgo JP, Westerhof N, Giolma JP, Altobelli SA. Effects of exercise on aortic input impedance and pressure wave forms in normal humans. Circ Res 1981 ; 48 : 334-43.

59 Siché JP, Mansour P, de Gaudemaris R, Mallion JM. Arterial compliance during exertion in hypertensive and normal subjects of the same age. Arch Mal Cœur Vaiss 1989 ; 82 : 1077-82.

60 Kingwell BA, Berry KL, Cameron JD, Jennings GL, Dart AM. Arterial compliance increases after moderate-intensity cycling. Am J Physiol 1997 ; 273 : H2186-91.

CHAPTER

Perspectives on clinical applications of pulse wave velocity

Large artery pathology is a major contributor to cardiovascular disease morbidity and mortality. The initiation and progression of these pathological alterations in large arteries is only partially understood. A distinct characteristic of these alterations is arterial stiffness. Increased arterial stiffness and PWV have been proposed as possible mechanisms in the initiation and/or progression and/or complications of atherosclerosis and cardiovascular risk factors and diseases. For more than 100 years, numerous clinical studies have been performed in healthy subjects and patients with different pathological conditions; they have highlighted the important role of arterial stiffness in pathophysiology as well as its possible implications in the management of these diseases. At the present time, the whole area of arterial stiffness is in a state of flux, which is reflected by a considerable and increasing number of publications on this field over recent years. Regarding future research in clinical applications of arterial stiffness, different aspects may be considered: technical developments, applications in pathophysiology, diagnosis, prognosis and therapy.

TECHNICAL DEVELOPMENT

Most of the devices used for measuring PWV were based on paper recorders and hand-held probes to detect various pulse signals: pressure, flow, diameter, volume, etc. Calculation of the time interval between the foot of the proximal and distal waves was usually made manually on the recorded paper; the distance between the two probes was measured directly over the skin. In the last decade, automatic computerised devices to measure the time delay between two pulse waves and to calculate PWV have become available. In order to facilitate the PWV measurement in the clinic, different parts of its determination may be improved, as described below.

• Use of a simple signal to detect pulse wave: at present, the most frequently used signals are pressure and flow signals detected using a mechanical piezo-electric or Doppler transducer. Other signals, easier to detect may facilitate, if suitable, the signal detection and recording procedure. In this regard, signals based on ultrasound, photoplethysmography and tonometry are under evaluation. Elsewhere, in order to facilitate the signal detection, probes, including several sensors, are under development. The principle of this multi-sensor probe is simple: the probe presents a large application surface which contains several sensors; the sensor corresponding to the best quality signal recorded is automatically selected. In order to avoid the use of a special device to handle the probes or the use of handheld probes, different variants of probes, using simple strips for maintaining their position, are under development.

• In order to facilitate PWV measurement, specifically designed small devices may be developed. Such dedicated devices may be completely independent or may be connected to any computer. Elsewhere, common cardiologic equipment, such as the ECG or echocardiograph, may include a complementary modulus for PWV measurement.

• Since arterial stiffness may be affected in a different manner in the various arteries, simultaneous measurements of PWV in different arterial pathways has to be proposed, at least in two different arteries. In fact, such simultaneous measurements will allow investigators to assess central and peripheral arteries, elastic and muscular arteries, or to perform bilateral recordings useful in some specific clinical situations.

• Measurement of the distance between the proximal and the distal probes needs to be improved in order to limit the range of errors. In the meantime, there is a need for consensus in the optimal distance measurements.

APPLICATIONS IN PATHOPHYSIOLOGY

A number of studies have described the major and minor determinants of PWV in different populations. Associations between PWV and a number of cardiovascular diseases have been reported. The role of PWV in different pathophysiological conditions has been shown. However, the initiation and progression of the alterations in large arteries is only partially understood. In fact, arterial stiffness may be important in the etiology and natural history of several cardiovascular outcomes. Therefore, the natural history of cardiovascular disease may be more accessible to study and perhaps better understood. In fact, most of the published studies to date have been cross-sectional and thus the antecedents of increased arterial stiffness are unknown. Prospective studies will assist in the determination of whether alterations in arterial stiffness precede the development of cardiovascular diseases or vice versa.

Genetic profiles can influence the vulnerability of the cardiovascular system; identification of genetic markers may be of major interest in the detection of high risk patients. Studies have shown associations between arterial stiffness and polymorphisms of some genes coding for proteins that are implicated in the cardiovascular regulation; moreover, some gene polymorphisms have been shown to influence the effects of antihypertensive drugs on blood pressure and large arteries. Since atherosclerosis and cardiovascular diseases are multifactorial and heterogeneous diseases, and considering the interactions between several polymorphisms of different genes, large population studies are needed. In fact, in order to evaluate the role of polymorphisms of several genes and their interactions on arterial stiffness, and to analyse their influence on the effects of cardiovascular therapy, wide clinical trials involving a large number of patients, and thus different polymorphisms of several genes, are still required.

The relationships between arterial stiffness and other cardiovascular parameters or risk factors have been described. The role of PWV as a determinant of more recently emergent markers, such as pulse pressure, heart rate, etc., and its role in some cardiovascular diseases such as heart failure, etc., and peripheral vascular diseases need further specific studies.

APPLICATIONS IN DIAGNOSIS

Numerous studies have shown associations between arterial stiffness and number of cardiovascular risk factors and diseases. Moreover, measurements of arterial stiffness may also serve as indicators of cardiovascular disease. Therefore, young adults who are at high risk could be identified before clinical cardiovascular complications develop. To progress in this field, there is a need for consensus in the optimal measurement and reporting of arterial stiffness.

• Choice of technique: use of techniques based on ultrasound, plethysmography, pressure transducer, etc.? Local or segmental distensibility?

• Choice of the parameter: there is a need for consensus on the chosen hemodynamic parameter: PWV, index normalised for age and blood pressure, stiffness index, isobaric distensibility or compliance?

• Choice of the artery: must measurements be performed on one or several arterial sites? Over one or different arterial points or over one or different arterial segments?

• Definition of normal values: may normal values be defined as those observed in normal patients, those observed as cut-off values from prognostic studies or those calculated from data obtained in different studies and population, in meta-analysis, etc.? May results be expressed as absolute values or by comparison to normal threshold using absolute or percentage values?

Furthermore, prospective studies are needed to determine whether alterations in arterial stiffness precede the development of cardiovascular diseases or vice versa. Analysis of the specificity and sensitivity values of arterial stiffness for the diagnostic evaluation of cardiovascular diseases and their complications need to be further evaluated.

APPLICATIONS IN PROGNOSIS

Studies have shown PWV as a marker of cardiovascular risk in hypertensive patients, and as an independent marker of all-cause and cardiovascular mortality in patients with end-stage renal disease. Longitudinal studies will make the natural history of cardiovascular diseases more accessible and perhaps better understood.

Evaluation of the prognostic value of arterial stiffness in a large population with and without known cardiovascular risk factors and/or diseases will help establish the role of arterial stiffness as an independent marker of morbidity and mortality, by analysing its specificity and sensitivity by comparison to other factors. Such determination of threshold values may allow young adults who are at high risk to be identified before clinical complications develop, thus the range of options for appropriate intervention at the individual level and in the general population could be expanded.

Longitudinal prospective studies are also needed in order to establish whether considering arterial stiffness and its reversion may improve patient prognosis.

APPLICATIONS IN THERAPY

Numerous pharmacological studies performed principally on hypertensive patients have shown that antihypertensive agents may improve arterial stiffness; this improvement was partially independent of blood pressure reduction. Elsewhere, studies have shown that antihypertensive agents may be differentiated by their effects on arterial stiffness. Moreover, evaluation of the arterial effects must take into consideration the arterial site, the drug doses used and the duration of the treatment. Taken together, these results show that there is a need for further pharmacological studies to evaluate the arterial effects of different dosages of various antihypertensive agents on at least two arterial segments (muscular and elastic) according to long-term treatment protocol. Such double-blind studies performed on a large number of patients will allow the comparison of the arterial effects of the different antihypertensive agents.

Although the arterial effects of some antihypertensive agents have been evaluated, very few studies have investigated the arterial effects of the treatments of the other cardiovascular risk factors. In fact, considering that the arterial wall is the site of all the cardiovascular risk factor complications, there is a need to evaluate the arterial effects of the different cardiovascular risk treatments.

Moreover, large clinical trials performed under similar conditions to our clinical practice are also needed in order to evaluate the ability of different treatment regimens to improve the physical properties of large arteries. To date, only one large-population clinical trial has been performed in hypertensive patients: the Complior® study. Further studies evaluating different treatment regimens in hypertensive patients are needed. Similar trials are also desirable in patients with diabetes or hypercholesterolemia to evaluate the arterial effects of different anti-diabetic or hypocholesterolemic regimen treatments.

Prospective studies designed to evaluate the arterial effects of non-pharmacological treatments of cardiovascular risk factors are also needed.

Finally, whether improvement or reversion of arterial stiffness improves the patient's prognosis needs to be confirmed by specific studies.

Thus, for more than 100 years, numerous case reports and clinical studies have been performed on healthy subjects and on patients with different pathological conditions. At the present time, the whole area of arterial stiffness is in a state of flux. Regarding future research, there is a need for numerous studies in the different clinical fields, from pathophysiology to therapy, and for consensus on the optimal measurement, reporting and interpretation of arterial stiffness should have top priority.

Key word index

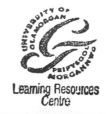

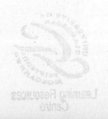